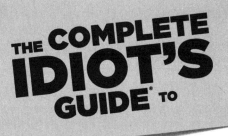

THE COMPLETE
IDIOT'S
GUIDE® TO

Boosting Your Immunity

D0840101

by Murdoc Khaleghi, MD, and Colleen Totz Diamond

ALPHA

A member of Penguin Group (USA) Inc.

ALPHA BOOKS

Published by Penguin Group (USA) Inc.

Penguin Group (USA) Inc., 375 Hudson Street, New York, New York 10014, USA • Penguin Group (Canada), 90 Eglinton Avenue East, Suite 700, Toronto, Ontario M4P 2Y3, Canada (a division of Pearson Penguin Canada Inc.) • Penguin Books Ltd., 80 Strand, London WC2R 0RL, England • Penguin Ireland, 25 St. Stephen's Green, Dublin 2, Ireland (a division of Penguin Books Ltd.) • Penguin Group (Australia), 250 Camberwell Road, Camberwell, Victoria 3124, Australia (a division of Pearson Australia Group Pty. Ltd.) • Penguin Books India Pvt. Ltd., 11 Community Centre, Panchsheel Park, New Delhi—110 017, India • Penguin Group (NZ), 67 Apollo Drive, Rosedale, North Shore, Auckland 1311, New Zealand (a division of Pearson New Zealand Ltd.) • Penguin Books (South Africa) (Pty.) Ltd., 24 Sturdee Avenue, Rosebank, Johannesburg 2196, South Africa • Penguin Books Ltd., Registered Offices: 80 Strand, London WC2R 0RL, England

International Standard Book Number: 978-1-61564-318-9
Library of Congress Catalog Card Number: 2013930720

15 14 13   8 7 6 5 4 3 2 1

Interpretation of the printing code: The rightmost number of the first series of numbers is the year of the book's printing; the rightmost number of the second series of numbers is the number of the book's printing. For example, a printing code of 13-1 shows that the first printing occurred in 2013.

Printed in the United States of America

Note: This publication contains the opinions and ideas of its author. It is intended to provide helpful and informative material on the subject matter covered. It is sold with the understanding that the author and publisher are not engaged in rendering professional services in the book. If the reader requires personal assistance or advice, a competent professional should be consulted.

The author and publisher specifically disclaim any responsibility for any liability, loss, or risk, personal or otherwise, which is incurred as a consequence, directly or indirectly, of the use and application of any of the contents of this book.

Most Alpha books are available at special quantity discounts for bulk purchases for sales promotions, premiums, fund-raising, or educational use. Special books, or book excerpts, can also be created to fit specific needs. For details, write: Special Markets, Alpha Books, 375 Hudson Street, New York, NY 10014.

Publisher: *Mike Sanders*

Executive Managing Editor: *Billy Fields*

Executive Acquisitions Editor: *Lori Cates Hand*

Development Editor: *Kayla Dugger*

Production Editor: *Jana M. Stefanciosa*

Book/Cover Designer: *Rebecca Batchelor*

Indexer: *Brad Herriman*

Layout: *Ayanna Lacey*

Proofreader: *Gene Redding*

Contents

Introduction

The immune system is a key component of your health. When you think of the immune system, you may associate it with preventing and fighting colds, but the immune system does so much more. From less serious respiratory infections and gastrointestinal viruses to more serious infections like meningitis, your immune system helps fight all types of illness.

Your immunity not only prevents infections, but can also make them far more tolerable. With a strong immune system, once you face an infection, you are far more equipped to fight similar infections in the future. And your immunity doesn't just fight infections; a healthy immune system has also been shown to reduce the risk of cancer and even cardiovascular disease.

Fortunately, you can boost your immunity using many techniques, such as keeping your vaccines up to date, washing your hands, reducing your stress, increasing your physical activity, and eating certain foods and supplements, to name a few. Many of these immunity boosters have been well studied, proven, and used successfully by millions of people, and the only side effects are increased energy, improved mood, and overall better health.

Congratulations on taking the first step to improving your immunity, your health, and your life.

How This Book Is Organized

This book is broken down into four parts:

Part 1, How Immunity Works, discusses the inner workings of the immune system and its effect on your overall health. This part talks about the many types of viral and bacterial infections your immune system fights. It also describes some of the problems you can experience when things go wrong with your immune system.

Part 2, Giving Your Immune System a Fighting Chance, provides the tools you need to assist your immune system, including vaccine schedules, ways to defend against catching an infection, exercise tips, and stress-reduction ideas.

Part 3, Immune-Boosting Foods, Vitamins, and Supplements, discusses which foods pack the most immune-boosting nutrients per calorie and the proper way to structure your food intake to keep your immunity in top form. It also covers what certain vitamins and supplements do and how they can help your immune system.

Part 4, Steps Toward a Healthier Life, contains 25 recipes made from nutrient-rich, immune-boosting foods. This part also gives you an action plan for ditching bad habits and adopting healthy ones.

Extras

Throughout the book, you'll come across helpful sidebars that will provide you with additional information:

DEFINITION

These sidebars include definitions of key terms throughout the text.

IMMUNITY ALERT

Be sure to check out these sidebars, which include health alerts and warnings against things that could negatively affect your immunity.

IMMUNE BOOSTER

These sidebars provide general information about immunity and provide tips on ways you can boost your immunity.

Acknowledgments

Murdoc Khaleghi, MD: I would like to thank my co-author, Colleen Totz Diamond. I would also like to thank our acquisitions editor, Lori Cates Hand; our editor, Kayla Dugger; and my agent, Steve Ross.

Colleen Totz Diamond: I would like to thank my co-author, Murdoc Khaleghi, for his expertise and insights throughout the project. Special thanks to Lori Cates Hand, whose confidence in this project was unwavering, and to Kayla Dugger, our editor, for her steady hand in shaping our manuscript into a book. I would also like to thank Kim Ross, MS, RD, CDN, who provided the recipes for the book, and Heidi Bonanno-Ogrisek, who inspired much of the information about the importance of exercise. Last, a special thank you to my husband, David Diamond, who supports me completely and almost inexplicably in these mad dashes to publication.

Trademarks

All terms mentioned in this book that are known to be or are suspected of being trademarks or service marks have been appropriately capitalized. Alpha Books and Penguin Group (USA) Inc. cannot attest to the accuracy of this information. Use of a term in this book should not be regarded as affecting the validity of any trademark or service mark.

How Immunity Works

Your immune system defends against many types of infections—viral, bacterial, and other, atypical ones. Each major part of your body also has its own specialized defense mechanisms. In this part, you see how the various layers of the immune system work together to protect your body from infection and disease, including cancer.

But sometimes all is not well with the immune system. Therefore, it's important to interpret correctly what it means to have a weakened immune system or an autoimmune disease so you can live your best life despite these handicaps, as you'll learn to do in this part.

Your immunity affects your overall health in profound ways. In this part, you see the critical role that acute inflammation plays in keeping you healthy—and the destructive results of chronic inflammation. You also find out how to improve your general health so you can boost your immune health. Your immunity is directly tied to your health, so any changes in your immunity affect your health—and vice versa.

Immune System Basics

Chapter

1

In This Chapter

- Your layers of defense
- The innate immune system
- The adaptive immune system
- The lymphatic system
- Anatomy of an infection

Your immune system fights infections that put your health at risk. One key to the immune system's success is it has many layers of defense. If an infection somehow gets past one of the layers, other layers step up to fight the infection.

In this chapter, you learn about these different layers of defense: the innate immune system, adaptive immune system, and lymphatic system. You also get an example of the immune system in action, after it is exposed to a virus.

How Does the Immune System Work?

The immune system defends the body against foreign substances and harmful organisms, also known as *antigens*, by creating an immune response. Sometimes the immune system reacts to substances that aren't harmful to the body, such as in allergic reactions or the rejection of transplanted organs. (Allergies are a common problem, and we will cover this topic in Chapter 3.)

DEFINITION

Antigens are foreign substances and pathogenic bacterial, viral, fungal, and parasitic organisms that elicit an immune response.

Before the immune system can create an immune response to eliminate an antigen, it must first recognize the antigen. The immune system can recognize millions of antigens and can remember antigens that it encountered previously, helping it build immunity, or resistance, to these types of exposures. When you have immunity to an antigen, your immune system recognizes and eliminates the antigen more efficiently.

Think of the immune system as a multilayered defense. The first and often overlooked layer of the immune system is the skin, which acts as a physical barrier to entry by antigens. The skin is part of your overall innate immune system, which acts against anything that isn't supposed to be there. Next is the adaptive immune system, which adapts to the specific exposure and stores it in its memory so that if it's ever exposed to the same thing again, it can respond even better. Next is the lymphatic system, which channels antigens to areas where the immune system is strongest. The combination of the way these layers work individually and the communication among them as a whole is what makes your immune system so remarkable.

Your Innate Immune System: It's in There

The innate immune system is your body's first line of defense against infection. The innate immune system works at the cellular level to consume and destroy antigens. The cells of the innate immune system don't pick and choose which pathogens they attack; they attack them all. They do, however, alert the cells of the adaptive immune system, which does selectively attack specific pathogens.

One of the ways you can tell that your innate immune system is active is by the presence of inflammation. Inflammation is what you get when your tissues swell, often turning red and feeling warm to the touch. This occurs when tissues become damaged or infected. Too much inflammation is not good, but inflammation does serve an important purpose. It leads to increased blood flow, which allows a rush of various immune factors to the area.

The complement system is part of the innate immune system. Its purpose is to amplify an immune response by calling a high amount of antibodies and certain immune cells to an affected area. The antibodies grab onto antigens, neutralizing and marking them for further attack. The complement system literally "complements" the rest of the immune process and represents an important layer of your body's immune defense.

Surface Barriers

To get into the body, antigens first must get past the body's surface barriers. The body's surface barrier is predominantly the skin, but also includes the tissues lining the body's internal passageways. Following are some basic facts on how each surface barrier works:

- The skin is generally a very effective barrier, though it can be penetrated by microcuts or tiny abrasions.
- The lining of the respiratory tract produces mucus and prompts sneezing or coughing to eliminate antigens from the nasal passageways and the lungs.
- The stomach defends against antigens found in food by destroying them in stomach acid.

If antigens pass through the body's surface barrier, they still have to find a way through the walls of your internal passageways. Your body has many ways to prevent that from happening.

Mucosal Immunity

The mucosal immune system works to maintain the health of your mucus membranes, which are the linings of the inside of your body that get exposed to the outside environment. This component of the immune system combats antigens that enter your tissues or find their way into your bloodstream through your digestive, reproductive, respiratory, and urinary tracts.

The mucosal immune system includes organs and nodes throughout your body that take the fight to the antigens. Each body system has its own features that work with the physical features of each organ system:

- Digestive tract: tonsils, appendix, intestinal lymphoid tissue, and gut flora
- Respiratory tract: adenoids, tonsils, and cilia
- Reproductive tract: cervical nodes and mucous
- Urinary tract: mucous and microflora

Bacterial flora can also assist the mucosal immune system. The next section covers these beneficial bacteria in more detail.

Normal Flora

Your skin and mucus membranes are home to a whole host of microorganisms, called *normal flora*. Many of these are considered beneficial; others are considered to be antigens. Normal flora are typically bacteria, but you have other types of non-bacterial microorganisms present that are also part of your normal flora.

Many of the normal flora can be harmful when not kept in check by your immune system. Here are some of the conditions that these bacteria can cause when permitted to grow in excess:

- Acne
- Colitis
- Colon cancer
- Dental problems
- Diarrhea
- Endocarditis
- Intestinal infections
- Meningitis
- Pneumonia
- Tonsillitis (strep throat)
- Urinary tract infections

Some normal flora are beneficial to human health. *Bifidobacterium bifidum*, for example, is found in the intestines of breastfed infants, where it boosts the infant's immunity. These bacteria are sometimes used in the manufacture of yogurts and are frequently incorporated into probiotics (see Chapter 12).

IMMUNITY ALERT

Taking antibiotics can kill beneficial bacteria, which can impair digestive functioning. To offset this effect, take probiotic supplements or eat yogurt that has live cultures.

Immune Cells

The immune system is host to a huge number of cells. Some of these cells attack any antigen they encounter regardless of type; others are more selective and attack just one type of antigen. To get the job done, the various types of immune cells work together, communicating through direct contact or chemical transmitters.

There are three main types of antigen-killing white blood cells: phagocytes, T cells, and B cells.

Phagocytes are large white cells that can engulf and digest foreign invaders—they literally eat them up. Phagocytes include the following cells:

- Monocytes, which circulate in the blood.
- Macrophages, which are found in tissues throughout the body. These cells secrete powerful chemicals that play a big role in activating T cells.
- Neutrophils, which circulate in the blood and move into tissues as needed. These cells contain granules filled with powerful chemicals that destroy pathogens and create inflammatory responses.

There are different types of T cells. Some T cells turn off or suppress immune cells. The main role of other T cells is to regulate the immune system. These cells are known as *helper T cells*. Like macrophages that have been exposed to antigens, these helper T cells activate other immune cells, including B cells and other T cells. Then there are T cells known as *killer cells*, meaning they kill other cells. Following are two types of killer T cells:

- Cytotoxic T cells directly attack any cells carrying foreign or abnormal molecules on their surfaces. They go after cells that have been infected by viruses or transformed by cancer.
- Natural killer cells don't need to recognize a specific antigen to launch their attack; they simply look for cells that lack the molecular structure typical of a normal cell.

The last of the main immune cells, B cells, works by releasing *antibodies* into the body. Antibodies cannot penetrate healthy cells, but they can launch a direct attack on antigens in the bloodstream. Because antibodies cannot penetrate healthy cells, they have a harder time fighting viruses that hide within cells.

> **DEFINITION**
>
> **Antibodies** are proteins used by your immune system to launch a direct attack on the antigens in your bloodstream.

The Adaptive Immune System: Adapt for Survival

The adaptive immune system remembers what the immune system has encountered in the past, so the next time you are exposed to the same antigen, your immune system works a lot more effectively against it. It's much more efficient than the innate immune response, but it also wouldn't be possible without the assistance of that system. This memory and increased immune effectiveness are the whole concept behind vaccines.

> **IMMUNE BOOSTER**
>
> Vaccines are considered the single greatest advance in the fight against infections and the most valuable immune booster in existence. They actually arouse your immune system, which is why some people get sick after vaccines. Through this, they strengthen your immune system's response to future infections.

So if the immune system remembers the antigens it encounters, you should never have the same illness twice, right? Well, not exactly. If you catch a cold, the adaptive immune system will recognize that cold virus and fight it off should you ever be exposed again to that exact same virus. The exact types of infections, however, often change. For example, the flu virus mutates, or changes, each year. In addition, hundreds of different cold viruses exist, so generally you get infected by a different cold virus each time you catch a cold.

The infections don't need to be the exact same for the adaptive immune system to be helpful, though. Many types of infections share cross-reactivity, or have similar components. Because of this, your immune system can better fight certain infections that are related to previous infections to which you have been exposed.

Cell-Mediated Immunity

Cell-mediated immunity is an immune response that fights antigens without using antibodies. Instead, it uses natural killer T cells, phagocytes, and antigen-specific immune cells and chemicals.

Cell-mediated immunity is most effective at defeating microbes that live within the cells of the human body, since antibodies cannot penetrate these cells. This immune response commonly removes virus-infected cells, but it defends against other threats as well, including cancer.

A healthy immune system not only decreases your chance of infections, but also benefits other aspects of your health, including decreasing your risk of cancer.

Humoral Immunity and Antibodies

Humoral immunity is an immune response carried out by antibodies. *Humoral* refers to the noncellular parts of the blood, including plasma and lymphatic fluid. As part of the humoral immune response, antibodies occurring in the humoral kill antigens and activate the complement immune system.

Certain B cells produce an antibody designed to defeat certain types of antigens, such as specific bacteria. Antibodies cannot penetrate cells, making it more difficult for them to fight viruses that hide inside cells, but they do fight antigens directly in the humoral fluid. Antibodies strengthen the performance of immune cells, and immune cells (B cells) produce antibodies.

Antibodies function by binding antigens and using this binding to surround and inactivate them or to bring them to cells that can finish off the antigen. In addition, when antibodies bind to antigens, they can bind to cells that release various factors to make your immune system even stronger.

Immune Memory

Memory cells, which are specialized B cells and T cells, are the basis of immune memory, a key aspect of the adaptive immune system.

The reason these cells are important is because it is impossible for your body to contain all the immune cells from every antigen exposure you have ever experienced. Therefore, it stores memory of these exposures in specific cells that then activate your entire immune system when necessary.

When your body encounters an antigen it has encountered in the past, your immune system activates the corresponding memory cells. That way, each exposure to an antigen produces a progressively stronger and faster immune response.

Having a faster and stronger response can help control infections before they cause serious damage. For example, many vaccines exist for deadly bacterial infections such as *Pneumococcus* or *Haemophilus influenzae*, so if those bacteria are ever truly encountered, they are dealt with by your immune system before they become harmful to you.

You have two types of immune memory:

- Passive immune memory lasts from a few days to several months. Passive immunity exists in infants, who share some immunity from their mother for a short time.

- Active immune memory lasts long term. Active immunity can be acquired by having an infection (which triggers B cells and T cells) and through vaccines.

IMMUNE BOOSTER

Because the flu virus changes every year, you should get a flu shot every year. One vaccination protects you for one year.

The Lymphatic System: Lymphing Along

To make your immune system as strong as possible, your body either tries to bring immune factors to antigens or alternatively tries to bring antigens closer to areas where the immune system is strongest.

This latter method is conducted by your lymphatic system, a combination of vessels, nodes, and tissues that filters antigens to where they can be best eliminated.

Lympathic Vessels

Like the circulatory system, your lymphatic system consists of vessels that travel throughout your body to all of your tissues. By reaching all of your tissues, the lymphatic system can help collect antigens from everywhere in your body to make sure the highest concentrations of immune cells can be used throughout your body, including places where there may not be as many immune cells.

Much of your lymphatic system is actually in parallel to your circulatory system, with vessels traveling together. This helps the lymphatic system collect fluid, as most fluid that travels through the lymphatic system (or lymphatic fluid) comes from fluid that's pushed out of the circulatory system. By being present nearly everywhere your circulatory system exists, it can collect fluid from throughout your circulatory system.

The lymphatic system processes approximately 15 percent, or about one seventh, of your immune system every day. In other words, your lymphatic system processes nearly your entire circulatory system every week.

IMMUNE BOOSTER

The circulatory system has a parallel system of lymphatic vessels that carry fluid to areas with high concentrations of immune cells.

Just as a blood vessel can be damaged, lymphatic vessels can be damaged by surgery or trauma, and such damage can cause swelling in the area because the lymphatic vessel cannot process the extra fluid. Also, valves exist in lymphatic vessels that help lymphatic fluid move through the system. As you age or due to gravity, these valves or lymph vessel walls can become progressively incompetent, which can also cause fluid leakage and swelling. Therefore, you can have swelling in a single arm or leg due to lymphatic vessel damage or swelling in both legs from poor lymphatic flow due to weak vessels or valves in the vessels.

Lymph Nodes

Though lymphatic vessels help transport lymph fluid, they tend to not directly fight antigens. Instead, they bring antigens to areas that are full of immune cells and therefore better equipped to fight antigens. These areas are known as *lymph nodes*, so named because they are spherical or ball-like junctions of lymph vessels.

Lymph nodes have extremely high concentrations of immune cells. When an antigen is brought to a lymph node in the lymphatic fluid, these immune cells are activated to destroy the antigen by releasing granules or surrounding it with antibodies.

When lymph nodes function optimally, they activate when they detect antigen exposure. This causes the lymph nodes to swell and explains why you can have ball-like swelling in areas of infection. These swollen lymph nodes are most commonly detected in the neck in upper respiratory infections, such as throat or sinus infections. Lymph nodes can also swell in other areas of infection or irritation, such as the groin, which has lymph nodes near the urinary tract and female reproductive tract. Lymph nodes can often be felt in the armpit, or axilla, with certain chest infections due to respiratory tract exposures.

Lymphoid Tissue

The immune fighters of the lymphatic system are not just present in the lymph nodes, but also in other areas of the body connected with that system. These other tissues that are full of immune factors are known as *lymphoid tissue*. These tissues can range from linings of mucosa, to condensed areas, to entire organs.

The intestines are lined with lymphoid tissue, considered to be one of the most important aspects of our immunity. You have so much lymphoid tissue because the intestines are constantly exposed to antigens in what you ingest. This lymphoid tissue works closely with the bacterial flora in your gut.

Other surfaces exposed to the environment have lymphoid tissue as well. There's a lot of lymphoid tissue in your throat, including your tonsils. This is why when you have an infection in your throat, your tonsils swell to fight the infection, similar to lymph nodes. This swelling can often cause discomfort, which many people believe is pain from the infection. In actuality, it is discomfort from your immune response. You can also see this with other immune responses, such as fever or a runny nose, where it is your immune response to infection that actually causes the discomfort of being sick.

The spleen is the largest condensed of area of lymphoid tissue, being an entire organ with extremely high concentrations of immune cells. Much of your lymphatic flow goes through the spleen in addition to the lymph nodes, creating another layer of strength in your lymphatic system. The spleen is not required, as sometimes due to trauma the spleen needs to be removed, but it is helpful. Those who have had their spleens removed are known to have a higher risk of certain infections, especially bacterial infections.

The Immune System from Start to Finish

The overall immune response varies somewhat by the type of infection, but viral infections involve nearly all the main aspects of the immune system. In this section, you will follow the immune system after it's exposed to a virus. By seeing what happens to a virus, you can better understand the various layers of the immune system.

Initial Exposure

The first aspect of any infection is the exposure. Different infections are transmitted by different means, with the most common being direct contact or the inhalation or ingestion of liquid secretions. Ideally, you can act to even decrease these exposures, but avoiding all exposures is impossible, so we will assume a virus managed to get on the surface of the body.

Innate Immunity

The first layer of the immune system is the skin, which protects you from most infections. The skin doesn't cover everywhere, but the lining of your respiratory and digestive systems offer a similar layer of protection. This layer is not impenetrable, though, as you can have microcuts and abrasions that allow exposures to penetrate through. The mucosal surfaces share a similar overall tightness and ability for small antigens to penetrate.

Your mucosal surfaces generally have lymphoid tissue, which exists in a thin layer under the skin. Therefore, many antigens have to immediately face this lymphoid tissue, giving your immune system another chance to prevent an infection from entering the body.

Should an antigen surpass the lymphoid tissue, it then enters the blood. Throughout the blood, various hunter cells travel with receptors; if those cells' receptors bind to anything they don't recognize, they initiate an immune response. Antigens can be recognized by these cells or get filtered into lymphatic fluid to reach lymph nodes or the spleen, which have high concentrations of immune cells.

Naive Immunity

Should the immune system be activated by lymphoid tissue, cells in the blood, or cells in lymph nodes, they all start activating a combination of cell-mediated and humoral immunity. Phagocytes such as macrophages will attempt to digest or destroy the antigen while releasing chemicals that tell your immune system to rush components to where the foreign exposure was identified.

T cells work to identify the specific type of exposure while attempting with B cells to provide an immune-specific response. Since there are different T cells and B cells for different types of antigens—and the amount of T cells and B cells for each antigen is rarely enough to handle the exposure itself—the cells work to clone so there are more of the appropriate type of cells and antibodies for the antigen.

IMMUNITY ALERT

Not all immune cells are appropriate for every exposure. The immune system selects the right cells to be cloned and brought to the antigen.

Some of these cells attack the antigen directly, some modulate how strong the immune response is, and some work to store a memory of the antigen should there be a similar exposure in the future. Most importantly, all of the cells signal each other to make sure there's the right balance of each for both now and in the future.

Immune Memory

Should you ever face an antigen that you have been exposed to before, either through a previous infection or from vaccines, certain cells are ready to act. As mentioned in the previous section, your naive immunity has cells to handle most types of antigens, but not very many of them, forcing them to be cloned during an exposure.

Because of immune memory, there are more of these cells when we have been exposed to a similar antigen before. All of our immune cells are intimately connected with other cells in determining the level of immune response, so if more of these cells exist, there will be a greater immune response.

This faster and stronger immune response will cause many infections to be destroyed before they have a chance to replicate themselves and cause bodily harm.

The Least You Need to Know

- The immune system has many layers of defense.
- Immune cells work together to adapt and increase the immune response to certain offenders.
- Immunity has memory, making future immune responses to the same exposure faster and stronger.
- The various components of your immune system work together to create the most effective response.

What Does Your Immune System Fight?

In This Chapter

- Viral infections
- Bad bacteria and atypical infections
- Common areas of infection

All day, every day (and night), your immune system fights various types of infection, including viral, bacterial, and fungal infections. The stronger your immune system, the more readily it can fight off these infections, effectively stopping them right at the front door. Each type of infection transmits in a slightly different way, but the defense is often the same: excellent hygiene and having a healthy immune system.

This chapter describes the various types of infection that commonly occur and some common areas of infection. We also provide some ideas on how you can give your immune system a boost and avoid getting sick.

Going Viral

Most infections are caused by viruses. Unlike infections caused by bacteria, viral infections don't respond to antibiotics, because viruses are not actually living organisms. They're just pieces of genetic material, DNA and RNA, that get inside healthy living cells and cause the cells to become sick.

Even with strong immunity, you're bound to get a viral infection every once in a while, as they are the most common type of infection—partly because they are so contagious and omnipresent.

IMMUNITY ALERT

When you are sick with an infection, it's important to know whether you are sick with a viral or bacterial infection. If you take antibiotics when you don't need them, you risk killing off the beneficial bacteria in your system. This can have detrimental effects on your health, including causing atypical bacterial infections or fungal infections and building antibiotic resistance. Therefore, in the future, you might get sick with bacterial infections that are harder to treat with antibiotics.

The following sections describe some of the more common viral infections you may encounter.

The Common Cold

You wake with a sore throat on Monday, and by Wednesday you have various symptoms of a cold—congestion, coughing, and sinus pressure, with possibly fever, fatigue, and body aches. Sometimes a cold settles in your head, and sometimes it settles in your chest. (If you're *really* lucky, it will settle in both places at the same time.)

The cold virus you catch eventually goes away because your immune system uses the mechanisms discussed in Chapter 1 to fight and build immunity to the virus, so your body builds some immunity to a cold virus every time you have it. The trouble is, the common cold isn't caused by the same virus every time you are infected. The common cold is caused by a range of viruses that cause similar upper respiratory symptoms. In fact, over 200 viruses have been implicated in the common cold, and these viruses are constantly mutating. Therefore, it's difficult to build an immunity to "the common cold," even though you can build immunity to certain types of it.

Since you can't build a full immunity to colds, it's smart to have a good defense. The best defense against catching a cold is to limit exposure with good hygiene. Prevent the spread of the virus by covering your nose and mouth when you sneeze and covering your mouth when you cough.

Viral Gastrointestinal Infections

Gastrointestinal infections are like having a cold in your stomach, with the infection located in the intestines. These are nearly always caused by viruses and why they are often referred to as a "stomach virus" or "stomach flu" or the even more nonspecific "stomach bug" (see Chapter 3 for more information about the flu virus).

The symptoms are well known—stomach cramping, diarrhea (often bloody in the less-common bacterial form), nausea, and vomiting. As with colds and most other types of infection, fever can also be present, as a fever is the body's response to infection and puts the immune system on overdrive. In other words, a fever can be a sign of a healthy immune system, but it can also be worrisome and discomforting to people with the fever.

Like most viruses, the most common cause of gastrointestinal viruses is person-to-person transmission of the virus (the most common methods of transmission are discussed in Chapter 6). When people contract gastrointestinal viruses, they often assume it was something in the food they have recently eaten. Food-borne illnesses are actually far rarer and tend to be more serious bacterial infections rather than viral infections.

> **IMMUNITY ALERT**
>
> Antibiotics aren't generally used to treat gastrointestinal infections, even when the infection is bacterial. Antibiotics can actually make the infection worse because they can kill the good bacteria in the gut.

The best way to treat gastrointestinal infections is to stay hydrated and treat the symptoms. Often, drinking frequent small sips of clear liquids is adequate to stay hydrated even if you're losing fluid through vomiting and diarrhea. Clear liquids are easier for the gut to quickly absorb, so even if you are losing some of what is ingested, a portion will still be taken in by the body. They also require less work for the stomach and intestines and are therefore less likely to cause increased irritation to the gastrointestinal system.

Occasionally, though, the vomiting and diarrhea can be so severe that further intervention is needed, such as medications. The most effective over-the-counter medication for diarrhea is Imodium. However, diarrhea is also a method of expulsion of the infection, so there are some concerns that anti-diarrheals like Imodium can extend the duration or severity of the illness. Like any intervention, the benefit of preventing dehydration has to be weighed against the potential risk.

For vomiting, certain prescription medications are very effective for decreasing nausea and vomiting. Some of these medications are available in suppository form or can be absorbed under the tongue so that even if the medication cannot be swallowed, it can be effective. If you become so dehydrated that you become weak and have a hard time functioning, you may require fluids intravenously (IV), because IV fluids are able to bypass the gut.

As with colds, the best defense for gastrointestinal infections is to wash your hands before and after eating, after using the bathroom, and after you shake hands with people, especially when the stomach bug is going around.

The Common Flu

Fever, chills, body aches, with a sudden onset of respiratory or gastrointestinal system problems—you're pretty sure you have the flu. Sometimes it's difficult to distinguish a common cold from the flu, and there is no perfect way to know other than testing. But the flu tends to be more severe, have higher fevers, and cause more diffuse symptoms. For example, while a cold is usually confined to the respiratory or gastrointestinal system, the flu may hit all these systems at once and cause greater overall lack of well-being through fatigue or muscle aches.

Unlike the over 200 viruses that can cause the common cold, the common flu is only caused by the influenza virus. A great advantage of this is the flu virus can actually be tested for, unlike trying to test for the hundreds of cold viruses. Like many viruses, though, this virus has several types and can mutate, so contracting the flu once does not mean you'll be immune for the rest of your life. However, because there's not as much variety as there is with colds, it's easier to build some immunity for a certain period of time.

For this reason, getting a flu shot each year greatly lessens the chance you'll get the flu—though it's not a guarantee. The flu virus changes, or mutates, rapidly. The vaccines for the flu are manufactured based on the preceding year's virus, which is usually close enough to the new virus to be effective. Every once in a while, however, the virus mutates unexpectedly, and the vaccination doesn't offer quite the level of protection it normally does. Still, even if you contract a different form of the flu, because of the cross-reactivity of the different viruses, the vaccine may decrease the duration and severity of the illness.

IMMUNE BOOSTER

You must repeat the vaccination each year for the flu shot to keep pace with the virus. Having previous vaccinations will confer some protection because of cross-reactivity, but staying up to date with vaccines is the most valuable form of flu vaccine protection.

The best defense against any flu is not to get it in the first place. Flu season lasts from October through March—the winter months, roughly—so practicing good hygiene and limiting your exposure are essential during those months. For years it was thought it was the cold weather that caused the flu, but it's actually due to the close quarters people maintain during colder weather that allows for greater transmission (see Chapter 6 for more on preventing or limiting exposure).

As a last defense, if you think you have the flu, don't hesitate to call your doctor. Your doctor may be able to prescribe antiviral medications such as Oseltamivir (Tamiflu) that if taken within the first 48 hours of infection will greatly lessen your symptoms. As with antibiotics, though, antivirals are only effective when given for the right infection and come with risks, so discuss with your physician whether the benefits of taking the medication outweigh those risks.

The Uncommon Flu

Certain years, an epidemic of a particularly severe virus occurs. These uncommon viruses are usually named for the species that originated the virus. Recent years have seen bird or avian flu, swine flu, and severe acute respiratory syndrome (SARS). Some of these are related to the influenza virus, like avian flu and swine flu (hence why they still have the flu name attached), while others like SARS are unique viruses that can cause flulike symptoms.

When epidemics such as this occur, many organizations work fever-ishly (no pun intended) to make a vaccine for the virus. Sometimes they're successful in doing so quickly, sometimes they're not, and sometimes they only make so much. In cases when there's a limited amount, the vaccines are often rationed to those who need it most, such as the elderly, young children, pregnant women, and those with especially weak immune systems and other diseases. When the epidemic is related to the flu virus, getting the flu virus vaccine can be of some benefit because of cross-reactivity, as it may decrease the chance of infection or lessen the severity or duration of symptoms.

As with the common flu, your main defenses against uncommon flu viruses are preventing transmission and, if the virus is transmitted, keeping your immune system in top shape.

Bad Bacteria and Atypical Infections

Even a healthy immune system can become overwhelmed by some bacteria. A weak immune system may be more susceptible to such infections. For example, a cut in the skin allows a portal of entry for skin bacteria. Antibiotics can kill healthy bacteria in the gut, occasionally allowing for an overgrowth of bad bacteria that are normally kept in check by other good bacteria. A very weak immune system also can open the door to atypical bacterial infections that don't infect healthy people but can wreak havoc in those with a weak immune system.

E. coli

Escherichia coli, or E. coli, is a bacteria normally present in the gut. Some strains of E. coli are actually considered beneficial, as long as the levels of all the bacteria in the gut are balanced. It's a certain strain of E. coli (0157) that's dangerous and can cause the symptoms of an E. coli infection. This more dangerous form can be transmitted as a food-borne illness. Beef, chicken, and pork are the usual foods that are recalled due to E. coli contamination, though it has been found in produce and dairy products as well. E. coli is also the most common bacteria in urinary tract infections because of the urinary tract's proximity to the colon.

The symptoms of an E. coli gastrointestinal infection are abdominal cramping and occasionally bloody diarrhea. The complications of an E. coli infection are anemia (low blood count) due to loss of blood and kidney damage or even kidney failure.

Unfortunately, no cure is available for E. coli gut infection, as antibiotics have not been shown to be effective. If you contract this illness, you must rest and stay hydrated. Also, although it sounds counterintuitive, avoid antidiarrheal medications when you have E. coli, as these medications slow down your digestive system while it's purging your body of the bacteria.

MRSA

All of us have bacteria that live on our skin. The most common of these bacteria are *Staphylococcus* and *Streptococcus*. Long ago, people could treat infections caused by these bacteria with basic antibiotics, like penicillin. Unfortunately, such common treatments led to the overgrowth of bacteria that were resistant to these antibiotics. Methicillin-resistant Staphylococcus aureus (MRSA) is a strain that's resistant to those common antibiotics and over time has become the predominant infectious skin bacteria.

The symptoms of a MRSA infection are dramatic and hard to stop:

- Abscesses—collections of pus under the skin
- Cellulitis—infection of the skin or fat and tissues immediately under it

- Infected follicles and boils—pus-filled infections on the skin's surface
- Sty—infection on the eyelid

IMMUNITY ALERT

If you suspect you have MRSA, seek immediate medical attention. Treatment involves specialized antibiotics and, if severe, may require hospitalization.

When MRSA advances beyond the skin and into the blood, it can spread to and possibly shut down major organs, a condition known as *sepsis*.

Though that's all very scary, it's also very real and speaks to the issue of antibiotic resistance. Having a strong immune system means that you require fewer antibiotics and therefore are less likely to promote the growth of antibiotic-resistant bacteria and develop antibiotic resistance in the future, which is good for you and society. Think of it this way—every time you avoid having to take antibiotics now, one more person can take those antibiotics safely in the future should he really need them.

C. diff

Clostridium difficile, or C. diff, is a common bacteria in the gut that is usually suppressed by other beneficial bacteria in the gut. If you have less of these good bacteria in your gut, such as when you take antibiotics, bacteria like C. diff become stronger.

C. diff infection causes gastrointestinal symptoms, such as stomach pain and diarrhea. All antibiotics can cause some stomach upset and diarrhea, but unlike many of these instances or gastrointestinal infections in general, C. diff infections will only progress without treatment using specialized antibiotics. This progression can lead to serious deadly bowel issues, including toxic megacolon, a potentially deadly loss of muscular tone in the bowel that can lead to spread of the infection or bowel rupture.

Like MRSA, it can only be treated with a few specialized antibiotics. Very few effective C. diff antibiotics can be given by mouth, so often people are hospitalized with these infections. The trouble is, the hospital is the most common place to pick up an infection.

Atypical Infections

As if your immune system doesn't keep busy enough fighting off viral and bacterial infections, it also tackles other types of infection and exposures. Keep in mind, your immune system doesn't attack something because it recognizes it as "Virus Number 1" (not technically); it attacks something because it recognizes the substance—whether it's a fungus, a parasite, or simply a speck of dirt—as not belonging in your body.

Yeast flourishes in warm, moist environments, so certain areas of the skin, vagina, groin, feet, and other areas (such as a baby's bottom, in the case of diaper rash) are the places commonly affected by yeast infection. Taking antibiotics increases the chance of yeast infection because antibiotics kill the bacteria that typically suppress yeast. This is just another reason why avoiding antibiotics when possible is a good idea.

The following are symptoms of a vaginal yeast infection:

- Intense itchiness
- Vaginal discharge
- Vaginal irritation

Treatment for a vaginal yeast infection is pretty straightforward. You can use over-the-counter topical medicines, such as Monistat, or see your doctor for a prescription treatment.

IMMUNE BOOSTER

Lessen your chances of getting a yeast infection when taking antibiotics by eating yogurt that has live cultures or taking probiotic supplements.

Yeast infections on the skin, such as diaper rash, jock itch, and athlete's foot, are generally easy to treat with topical ointments, either prescribed by your doctor or via at-home remedies.

Fungal infections are caused by fungi that are more complex forms of yeast, but the end result is the same: a red skin rash that burns and is intensely itchy. Like yeast infections, fungal infections flourish in warm, moist areas.

Parasites most commonly affect the gastrointestinal tract, causing the symptoms of gastrointestinal infection described previously in this chapter. You can get parasites from water—especially internationally due to poorer hygiene in some countries—undercooked meat, and even your pets.

The reason you can get parasites when you travel internationally while people who live abroad don't tend to get these infections as easily is simply because of the fact that you don't build immunity to these parasites when you are young. It makes sense that you don't have immunity to these parasites: you live in a more sterile environment, so you don't build memory and antibodies to these infections (as discussed in Chapter 1).

A common parasite in the United States is toxoplasmosis, which you can catch from cat feces. Toxoplasmosis can cause flulike symptoms or no symptoms at all. Most people with healthy immune systems will fight off the infection with little difficulty, while those with an impaired immune system can develop severe infections. Pregnant and nursing mothers should avoid changing cat litter, however, as toxoplasmosis can be quite serious if passed on to newborn babies. Proper hygiene around the litter box—covering your mouth and nose and washing your hands well, up to the elbows—provides adequate protection. Cats catch the parasite by eating infected mice, so if your cat doesn't go outside, it most likely won't carry the parasite. Also, the parasite doesn't live indefinitely in your cat.

Where It Hurts

Infections can be thought of not only as the contagion itself, but also the part of the body that is most affected. Every part of the body is affected differently by infections and manifest in various symptoms. By knowing how the systems in your body are affected, you can learn how to maximize your immunity against such infections and improve your overall health.

IMMUNE BOOSTER

Many infections end in –*itis,* which simply means "inflammation of [that area]." Therefore, bronchitis is inflammation in the bronchi, or upper airways, of the lungs. Of note, as –*itis* refers to inflammation and not infection—and there are many different causes of inflammation—you can have an –*itis* without necessarily having an infection. However, if you have an infection, there tends to be inflammation associated with it.

Lungs

The most common infections in the lungs are bronchitis in the upper airways and pneumonia in the lower airways. These lung infections occur when bacteria travels from the air or from your sinuses or throat into the lungs, since the lungs are very exposed. Pneumonia is common and can be very serious. It tends to come on quickly and often as a complication of an existing viral upper respiratory infection that has already impaired immune function in the lung. As you recall from Chapter 1, the lung has its own mechanisms and immune cells to fight infection, so it's important to have a strong immune system in the lungs to prevent viral infections that increase susceptibility to more serious bacterial infections. You can strengthen your immunity against lung infections with simple methods such as deep breathing and physical activity, which promote oxygenation of immune cells and tissue and lymphatic flow in the lungs.

Since pneumonia is most commonly caused by specific bacteria, certain vaccines can decrease the chance of contracting pneumonia as well as its severity, similar to the flu vaccine. If you are 65 or older or have an immune deficiency (see Chapter 3), it's recommended that you get vaccinated for pneumonia. The pneumonia vaccine lasts for five years. By then you will need to be revaccinated to boost your immune memory to the bacteria, which can slowly fade over time.

Throat

We all have bacteria in our throat, but sometimes our throat can get infected with a virus or by bacteria. The most common bacteria that infects the throat is known as *Streptococcus pyogenes*, otherwise known as group A strep or just strep for short.

IMMUNITY ALERT

Strep infections are treated with antibiotics. Left untreated, these infections can do long-term harm to your heart and kidneys.

Strep is easily tested for with a throat swab, though this test is not perfect. The swab will miss strep about 10 percent of the time, and about 1 in 5 people is considered chronic carrier of strep and will have a positive test even when not suffering an active infection. There are swabs with greater accuracy, but these can take days to produce results, unlike the few minutes the more common but less accurate swabs do. Fortunately, a physician can find other signs of a strep infection during a physical exam, so between that and the swab, your doctor can make the appropriate decision on antibiotics.

Interestingly, strep improves regardless of antibiotic treatment, though antibiotics have been shown to decrease the duration and severity of symptoms. The main reason antibiotics are often pre-scribed for strep is because an untreated infection has been shown to affect numerous body systems, including the heart and kidneys.

Strep remains susceptible to penicillin, as for certain physiological reasons strep hasn't developed a resistance to this common antibiotic.

Regardless, antibiotics are still overused for throat infections, often because physicians know patients are often seeking them. Make sure to ask your physician about how convinced he is that you have a true strep infection and how he thinks the antibiotics will affect that infection.

If you have a viral pharyngitis, all you can do is treat the symptoms. Your doctor may recommend specific lozenges and sore throat soothers, such as those that contain menthol (a topical anti-inflammatory) or benzocaine (a topical anesthetic). Pain relievers like acetaminophen (Tylenol), ibuprofen (Motrin), or naproxen (Aleve) may help relieve both the discomfort and any fever.

IMMUNE BOOSTER

To relieve pain from a sore throat, gargle saltwater. Dissolve 4 teaspoons of salt in a small glass of warm water and gargle deep in your throat.

Sinuses, Bronchi, and Ears

We all have bacteria in our throat and sinuses, and these bacteria can travel to the ear canals, sinuses (which are various pockets in the skull), and the upper airways or bronchi.

Most sinusitis and bronchitis infections are viral and don't require or respond to antibiotics. Knowing whether you have a viral or bacterial infection can be tricky, as the objective tests to distinguish these can be quite complicated and are not typically performed. As a general guideline—but with many exceptions—viral infections will be temporary (such as for a few days), but bacterial infections will persist and worsen. You should have approximately two weeks of persistent symptoms of sinusitis or bronchitis before starting antibiotics—sometimes longer. Though there are risks to lack of treatment—including developing abscesses, blood clots, and pneumonia from spread of the infection—such complications often take months of progression of the infection.

Ear infections are far more common in young children due to the shape of the ear canal when young, making it easier for bacteria to enter. As with sinusitis and bronchitis, many of these infections are viral. Also like those infections, the risk of ear infections is they can spread to other parts of the head, causing more serious infections. This spread can happen faster in younger children with weaker immune systems, so there's a lower threshold to treat these infections with antibiotics in young children. (We will discuss how to boost immunity in young children in Chapter 5.)

Within the last two decades, vaccines have been developed for the bacteria in ear infections that tend to be the most virulent (see Chapter 6 for more about these vaccines). Because of this, there is less risk of serious harm from an ear infection and more of a movement to delay antibiotic treatment to see if symptoms improve and antibiotics are no longer required.

Urinary Tract

Urinary tract infections (UTIs) are the most common true bacterial infections. UTIs are far more common in women because of their shorter urethra, making it easier for bacteria to travel up the urethra into the urinary tract. Bacteria that cause UTIs are typically coliform bacteria, or bacteria that live in and exit the colon, due to its proximity to the urinary tract.

The following are symptoms of a UTI:

- Blood in urine
- Burning during urination
- Lower belly pain
- Urgency to urinate

As people get older, UTIs can cause other more systemic symptoms, such as weakness and mental disturbances, due to older people having a weaker immune system. So small infections can easily spread and cause symptoms throughout the body.

Bacterial UTIs can be tested for with a simple urine test, and any uncertain cases can be grown in a laboratory culture to see if there is bacterial growth. The treatment for bacterial UTIs is antibiotics. Certain over-the-counter medications like pyridium (azole) act as a bladder anesthetic, which can temporarily decrease the discomfort until the antibiotics take effect.

IMMUNITY ALERT

Common STDs like gonorrhea and chlamydia can be confused with UTIs, as they produce similar symptoms. They are best distinguished with urine tests and bacterial swab testing.

Digestive Tract

Gastrointestinal infections, specifically in the small and large intestines, are very common. They are most often viral and spread through direct contact, though bacterial infections do occur and most commonly spread through food-borne illnesses. Though there are seriously harmful bacteria such as E. coli 0157, many bacterial infections act similarly to viral infections, with nausea, vomiting, abdominal cramping, and diarrhea (though bloody diarrhea is seen more commonly in bacterial infections). Bacterial infections are often treated similarly to bacterial infections, as these infections tend to be self limited and don't require antibiotics. Therefore, the main treatment is symptomatic, meaning you will be given medicines for nausea, diarrhea, and discomfort caused by these infections. In addition, taking in as much fluids as possible will help prevent dehydration.

Meninges

Meningitis is an uncommon but extremely dangerous infection in the area around the brain known as the meninges. Although uncommon, the bacterial form of meningitis is deadly and therefore should be taken very seriously. Vaccines have decreased the incidence of bacterial meningitis markedly, but it still occurs. Viral meningitis can have serious outcomes, but most often it resolves without serious complications. The only way you can know whether you have the viral or bacterial form of the infection is to see your doctor, who will test the spinal fluid via an invasive procedure called a *lumbar puncture*, otherwise known as a *spinal tap*.

The symptoms of severe meningitis are as follows:

- Fever
- Photophobia (difficulty viewing light)
- Severe headache
- Stiff neck

Often, people get a headache when they develop a fever, so simply the combination of fever and a headache don't necessarily require testing for meningitis, especially considering the risk of testing.

The symptoms are different for children under age 2. They are as follows:

- Bulge on the soft spot of the head (for a baby)
- Constant crying
- Difficulty feeding
- Excess sleepiness or sluggishness
- High fever
- Irritability
- Rigidity or stiffness of the neck or body
- Seizures

As with other infections, one of the most effective ways you can prevent meningitis is to make sure you and your children receive the appropriate vaccines.

The Least You Need to Know

- Most infections are either viral or bacterial, the key difference being that bacterial infections respond to antibiotics, while viral infections most respond to your own immunity.
- Antibiotics can have harmful side effects, including killing good bacteria that suppress other infections and promoting antibiotic resistance.
- The key defense to all infections is prevention of transmission, which will also decrease transmission, duration, and severity of most illnesses.

When Good Immune Systems Go Bad

In This Chapter

- Living with a weakened immune system
- Dealing with an overactive immune system
- Taking care of yourself so you can live your best life

The immune system is a complex and efficient system that, when working properly, ensures good overall health. However, some people don't have an immune system that functions properly. In some people, the immune system is weakened either by a genetic condition or a disease. In others, the immune system is overactive, causing allergies or autoimmune diseases.

This chapter describes some of the main features of these conditions and offers ideas on ways you can improve your health despite the limitations they impose.

Too Little Immunity

When you are sick, your immune system is weakened because it's busy fighting off the infection plaguing your system. As you ward off and recover from your cold or flu or stomach virus, your immune system creates memory cells so that the next time you encounter the same sickness, your body's response is more efficient. If everything works properly, you'll have less of a chance of contracting a similar illness, or you'll have an easier time fighting it off.

Unfortunately, your immune system doesn't always work properly. Some people develop or are born with a very weak immune system. This is called an *immune deficiency*. As you can imagine, this affects the immune system's ability to fight all sorts of infectious diseases and even cancer.

> **DEFINITION**
>
> An **immune deficiency** is when the immune system is weakened or completely crippled, increasing the risk of infection.

Causes of Immune Deficiency

Some people are born with a weak immune system. These people typically have genetic disorders, including deficiencies in antibodies such as agammaglobulinemia, immunoglobulin A (IgA) deficiency, and common variable immune deficiency. However, this is a comparatively rare cause of weakened immunity.

Most people who have a chronically weak immune system get the condition from taking medications designed to suppress the immune system. A doctor may give a person these medications to do the following:

- Treat allergies or asthma
- Manage an autoimmune disease (a condition in which the immune system is overactive)
- Treat cancer
- Prevent the body from rejecting new tissue after an organ transplant

The most common medications known to suppress the immune system are steroids, such as prednisone. These medications work by suppressing inflammation, including healthy inflammatory responses by your immune system. This induced weakness of the immune system makes people more susceptible to minor and severe infections.

Other medications are even stronger. Chemotherapy, for example, is used to kill cancer cells. Unfortunately, the only way it can kill the right cells is to kill some healthy cells, too, including immune cells.

Many diseases directly or indirectly weaken the immune system. Many types of cancer, particularly those of the bone marrow and blood cells (leukemia, lymphoma, aplastic anemia, multiple myeloma), and certain chronic infections directly weaken the immune system.

Immune deficiency is also the primary effect of acquired immunodeficiency syndrome (AIDS), caused by the human immunodeficiency virus (HIV). HIV directly infects the immune system's T helper cells and also impairs other immune responses directly.

Risks of Weakened Immunity

Besides getting sick more often and longer, people with very weak immune systems are at risk of catching *opportunistic infections*. Many of these opportunistic infections exist, including highly atypical bacteria, unusual viruses, and fungi.

 DEFINITION

Opportunistic infections are infections that don't normally pose a threat but become active when a person's immune system is weakened.

That's how HIV hurts you. The virus itself doesn't cause any symptoms, but because it suppresses your immune system, it opens your body up to all sorts of infections, including infections that don't affect people with healthy immune systems.

The infections become so common for people with very weak immune systems that they often have to take preventative, or prophylactic, medications against infections they are more likely to contract because of their weakened immune systems. But these medications can have harmful side effects.

There is a silver lining. If you have a very weak immune system, you are not powerless to help yourself. Working closely with your doctor to take precautions against getting infections and making customized, healthy lifestyle adjustments can pave the way to living a fulfilling life. Furthermore, many of the interventions in this book, while not able to completely restore immunity that is highly impaired by medications or disease, can still benefit your weakened immune system.

Increased Risk of Cancer

In addition to atypical infections, another problem with having a very weak immune system is an increased risk of certain types of cancer. In fact, it was through people with a severely weakened immune system that we learned the immune system, in addition to preventing infections, also helps prevent and suppress cancer. A healthy immune system can help recognize abnormal (cancerous) cells and eliminate them before they mature. But a weak immune system is unable to respond quickly or effectively enough, and cancer cells mature and multiply, eventually overwhelming the immune system.

Since we know a severely weakened immune system significantly increases the risk of cancer, it is logical to assume that even a healthy immune system that's not functioning optimally could increase risk of cancer as well. Therefore, a benefit of boosting your immunity is not only a decreased risk of various infections and a better ability to fight those infections, but a decreased risk of cancer as well.

Knowing that the immune system helps suppress cancer cells, it's clear that the stronger your immune system, the lower your risk of cancer. But what if you already have cancer?

When the immune system is unable to eradicate cancerous cells, medications, surgery, chemotherapy, and radiation are conventional treatments, but many of these treatments can impair the immune system further. Therefore, in those who do have cancer and require these sorts of treatments, it is essential to do whatever they can to improve their immunity.

In fact, now that more is known about the relationship between the immune system and cancer, immunotherapy is commonly used to boost the immune system. One of the best boosts to the immune system, though, is that which you can produce yourself through many of the interventions—from lowering your stress levels to eating an immune-boosting diet—discussed throughout this book. These interventions support your natural immunity and often have positive rather than negative side effects for other aspects of your health.

Cancer is seen in a whole new light today compared to how it was seen just 10 or even 5 years ago. There's so much people can do to improve their health today that they didn't know years ago, and more ways are learned every day. Don't ignore your well-being if you're given a cancer diagnosis, or any diagnosis, for that matter. Give life your all, and you stand to benefit.

IMMUNE BOOSTER

Immune-boosting habits can help ease the pain of an immune-related disease or even cancer. Following good nutrition, reducing stress, and getting exercise are proven aids to immunity. You may also consider joining a support group or participating in energy therapies, such as reiki and healing touch.

Is There Such a Thing as Too Much Immunity?

In some people, immune systems can actually be *too* strong. An immune system is too strong when either it attacks your innate healthy tissue that it usually ignores or overresponds to a foreign antigen so that the body experiences negative effects that outweigh the benefit of the response.

This generally is due not to healthy immune-boosting activities, but to genetics or hypersensitivities to certain things in the body or environment. Therefore, boosting your immunity through the practices in this book will not worsen these diseases because our recommendations are for boosting your natural immunity, while these diseases are unnatural.

Allergies

Allergies are essentially the immune system on overdrive. When you have an allergy, your immune system has a heightened sensitivity or excessive reaction to something that is usually not harmful, such as dust, mold, pollen, pet dander, and particular foods. These substances are called *allergens*.

> **DEFINITION**
>
> An **allergy** is a sensitivity of the immune system to a substance that is normally harmless, called an **allergen.** Allergens include dust, mold, pollen, pet dander, and certain foods.

When you are exposed to something that your body considers an allergen, you have an allergic reaction. Allergic reactions are inflammatory immune reactions caused when the immune system releases histamines and other substances in response to exposure to an allergen.

These are some common allergy symptoms:

- Anaphylaxis—a dangerous whole-body reaction, often characterized by the allergic person's throat "closing" and blood vessels dilating, causing a severe blood pressure drop
- Asthma—coughing, chest tightness, and shortness of breath
- Diarrhea—usually from food allergies
- Eczema—an itchy, scaly rash
- Hay fever—sneezing; coughing; runny nose; itchy, watery eyes; and sinus headache
- Hives—an itchy rash
- Stomach upset—usually from food allergies

With such varied symptoms, how can one treatment address them all? Well, one approach is to use several treatments to treat many symptoms—for example, antihistamines, decongestants, and nasal sprays all work for different aspects of hay fever. For more severe and persistent allergies, your doctor may want to prescribe something more potent to ease your symptoms, such as steroids. The problem with medications such as steroids is though they decrease the excessive reaction, they impair your healthy immune reaction as well. Therefore, if you need to take steroids, boosting your body's natural immunity becomes even more essential.

 IMMUNITY ALERT

Anaphylaxis is an emergency characterized by swelling of the tongue or throat, trouble breathing, and low blood pressure. If you are experiencing these symptoms, call 911 immediately.

The best way to address allergies, however, may be to treat the root of the problem, rather than simply the symptoms. This sort of treatment focuses on your immune system.

The first thing you need to do is find out what precisely is causing your allergies. Your doctor can perform any number of tests to make this determination, including a variety of skin tests; blood tests; or, in the case of food allergies, an elimination diet (eliminating and reintroducing suspected food allergens from your diet to determine which causes a reaction).

Once you know what's setting off your immune system, you can work to desensitize it to each allergen. Your doctor typically does this by administering injections that contain some of the allergen. You return for a round of injections over a set period of time, with the amount of allergen increasing each time. As the amount of the allergen increases, the immune system builds a tolerance to the allergen—and no longer responds with an allergic reaction.

By understanding and anticipating what may be causing allergic reactions, you can avoid having to be on immune-suppressing medications and therefore offer a boost to your own natural immunity.

Other Hypersensitivities

Asthma is an immune response that is associated with wheezing and being breathless. Asthma is essentially an allergic reaction of the lungs. An asthma attack—wheezing and being breathless, for a mild attack—is usually caused by a trigger, such as exposure to an infection, allergen, cold air, exercise, or even stress. Of these, an infection is one of the most common causes; therefore, by supporting your immunity so that you have fewer respiratory infections, you can have fewer asthma exacerbations.

IMMUNITY ALERT

Asthma can be serious, so if you think you have it, you should see your doctor to discuss treatment options to prevent and not just treat flares.

Another common hypersensitivity is *eczema*, which is essentially an allergic reaction in the skin. The skin can be very itchy and develop red hives or plaques that have a discomforting feel and appearance.

The treatments for asthma and eczema are similar to the treatments for allergic reactions, except more focused on the part of the body where it is occurring. For asthma there are more inhaled treatments, and for eczema more topical skin treatments.

These sorts of hypersensitivities can be hereditary. Your genes determine not just whether you have hypersensitivity but how severely you have it. Another major factor in the degree of these hypersensitivities is when and how you were exposed to the things that cause these reactions, especially when you were young. In fact, these exposures at a young age are an essential part of your overall immune health.

Early in life, your body collects data and builds memory cells that will direct your immune system's reaction to substances when you are an adult. For some substances, your body habituates, or learns, that it's okay to be exposed to them. When your body habituates to a substance, it doesn't produce a reaction to that substance later. For other substances, you get sensitized, which means you have more severe reactions later in life.

For example, if you are raised in a sterile environment with very limited exposures, it's far more common to have allergic reactions later in life. The body perceives regular parts of the environment as novel and foreign and has an excessive reaction to them. Contrastingly, if you are exposed to certain foods too early in life, your body is not prepared for them, and you have reactions to them that increase later in life.

Scientists are constantly learning which exposures are helpful and which are harmful when young, but here are some general rules. During the first 3 months of age, immune systems are very weak, so it is helpful to keep young children away from contaminants and those who are ill. After that, children form much of their immunity from exposures, so children spreading various viruses and germs around are less serious, though it is still worth practicing basic hygiene. (Food exposures are discussed in a later section.)

Autoimmune Disease

Autoimmune disease is a condition where the immune system is overactive and actually attacks the body itself because it recognizes some of the body's own tissues as foreign. Autoimmune disease is typically genetic. That is, you can't catch autoimmune disease; you're born with it. When you have an autoimmune disease, your immune system attacks something valuable in the body, such as certain organs, causing them to fail.

> **DEFINITION**
>
> **Autoimmune disease** is a condition where the immune system is overactive and attacks the body itself, usually targeting particular organs, depending on the specific disease.

People with autoimmune disease often need to be on medications that suppress the immune system, such as steroids like prednisone or other stronger medications. These medications have many harmful side effects—most importantly, making the immune system weaker—which cause all the risks of an impaired immune system and would greatly benefit from boosting your natural immunity.

The following are some well-known autoimmune diseases:

Addison's disease occurs when a person's adrenal glands are damaged and have reduced function as a result of an immune response.

Celiac disease affects the small intestine. This disease is caused by a sensitivity to gluten, a substance included in most grains and other foods.

Crohn's disease occurs when the immune system fails to distinguish between harmless or beneficial cells or bacteria and harmful substances. It causes inflammation throughout the digestive tract.

Graves disease causes the thyroid gland to work overtime, called *hyperthyroidism*.

Hashimoto's disease involves chronic swelling of the thyroid gland, which may be visible as an enlarged neck or goiter. The result is reduced thyroid function, called *hypothyroidism*.

Multiple sclerosis occurs when the immune system attacks the body's nervous system. Symptoms vary among people who have the disease and can affect many parts of the body.

Psoriatic arthritis includes many of the symptoms of both rheumatoid arthritis (inflammation of the joints and surrounding tissues) and psoriasis (a skin condition involving red, scaly patches, usually around the elbows, knees, and scalp).

Rheumatoid arthritis (RA) involves inflammation of the joints and surrounding tissues, as well as other organs. Joints may become less mobile and possibly deformed as the illness progresses.

Systemic lupus erythematosus (SLE) is marked by chronic inflammation, generally affecting the skin and joints. As the disease progresses, the kidneys, brain, and other organs may be affected.

Ulcerative colitis is a chronic inflammatory condition that involves the large intestine, or colon. This disease occurs when the immune system attacks harmless or beneficial cells or bacteria.

All of these autoimmune conditions are treated with medications, most commonly immune-suppressing medications. Treatment for a few, such as those affecting the thyroid gland, may involve radiation or surgery. If you have celiac disease, you must avoid all food that contains gluten (mostly wheat and other grains).

The important thing to remember about autoimmune diseases is that if you follow your treatment plan and live a healthy, immune-boosting lifestyle, you can still live a fulfilling life despite being on immune-suppressing medications. You may still have a weaker immune system than you would if you weren't on these medications, but you will feel better than you would have otherwise—stronger and happier—if you take the best possible care of your health.

Food Intolerances

Food intolerances represent a significant type of autoimmune reaction. You have a significant amount of lymphoid tissue in your gut, and based on genetics and early exposures, your body can have an immune reaction to various foods. The most well-known food that causes a reaction is gluten, but many others can cause everything from severe allergic reactions (such as some people have with peanuts) to minor symptoms such as diarrhea and upset stomach.

Certain foods can be pro-inflammatory, while others are anti-inflammatory, which then has subsequent effects on the immune system.

 IMMUNITY ALERT

Food sensitivities can cause anaphylaxis, which is a medical emergency. Common foods that cause this reaction are peanuts and shellfish.

The foods you are exposed to at an early age can significantly impact your food intolerances or allergies later in life. Since the knowledge of when certain foods should be eaten is constantly evolving, parents should discuss these recommendations with their pediatricians and not expose their children to certain foods earlier than recommended.

How You Help Yourself

Genetics play a role in determining the strength of your immune system, but you can do a lot to bridge the gap between your genetic makeup and good immune health, too. The better you take care of your overall health, the stronger your immunity will be and the less likely you will be to get infections. Not only is this good just because you'll feel better in the short term, it also benefits your long-term health.

Your immune system and infections are intimately tied with most other aspects of your health. Here are a few examples:

- One of the risks of being sick frequently is that you can develop infections that persist chronically, such as bronchitis, sinusitis, or colitis.

- Some infections can cause lasting harm to your body. For example, strep throat can cause kidney problems and heart issues.

- Many infections have long-term, destructive effects on tissues. For example, pneumonia destroys lung tissue, and meningitis can cause hearing and nerve damage.

- Inflammation contributed to by infection and other factors has been associated with heart disease, cancer, dementia, and other chronic diseases.

The good news is that although infections come with risk, you can do a lot to protect yourself and the people around you from getting sick in the first place.

At the top of the list is to take care of yourself. Getting proper nutrition, exercising, and making good lifestyle choices all boost your immunity—which lessens your chances of getting sick and reduces your risk of long-term health problems. Taking care of your own immunity also lessens the chance that you'll pass infection along to someone else.

For example, staying active with moderate exercise several times a week has all sorts of health benefits. It elevates your mood, improves your heart health, and boosts your immunity. Unfortunately, when you are continually sick with infection, or if you suffer from a condition such as rheumatoid arthritis that causes pain, staying active can be difficult.

Being sedentary is a major risk factor for many diseases, such as heart disease and cancer. Indeed, being sedentary is associated with worse cholesterol, higher blood pressure, and even a shorter life span. Luckily, small changes reap big rewards in this area, and the rewards are cumulative. That is, the more activity you introduce, the more you'll be able to take on—and the greater the health benefits.

The following sections offer some ideas for ways you can diminish your risk of infection. If you live with a weak or overactive immune system, taking this direction will also help you live a more satisfying life. You will feel better all around than you would have otherwise.

Changing the World by Changing Yourself

Good health is a cornerstone of good living. If you have good health, you have more energy and are more productive. If you aren't sick, you can spend more time with your loved ones. You feel better, and you don't need to worry about passing along any contagious infections. At work, you are more focused and able to accomplish more, which can open the door to success you might not have known otherwise. So remember, decreasing infections is one of the most effective ways you can increase your time and energy at work and at home.

When you take steps to improve your immunity and your overall health, others pick up on your positive habits. Then, in turn, the people around them may pick up on their positive habits. Every person makes a difference in helping keep every other person healthier and less likely to spread disease. Oh, you'll always have to deal with the people who come to work sick. Hand them a tissue, and use a hand sanitizer after shaking their hand.

One aspect of how your own immunity affects others is *herd immunity*. Herd immunity is how a society, through our children and person-to-person contact, develops a common immunity to certain diseases. This is why it benefits everyone to get vaccinated and participate in other immune-supporting practices. Essentially, doing so decreases the risk for everybody.

DEFINITION

Herd immunity is how a society develops a common immunity to certain diseases. Vaccinations can play a role in developing herd immunity.

The most important way to prevent the spread of infection is to wash your hands—after you use the restroom, before you eat or prepare food, after you walk the dog, and anytime your hands have been exposed to germs. Now, you don't have to go crazy. Being a germaphobe isn't good, either—you don't want to forfeit resistance to your environment that constantly challenges and builds your immunity. If you do that, you'll get sick *more* often. But use common sense. After you shake hands with a lot of people, wash your hands or use a hand sanitizer.

The other thing to consider is that by taking care of your immunity, you're not only taking care of yourself. When you are sick, you can spread infection to others.

Have you ever tried to figure out who exactly gave you a cold? You usually have a handful of suspects, and you rarely feel sympathetic toward them. Of course, colds are spread person to person, but they are also very contagious. It's reasonably impossible to know exactly who gave you a cold. But when the sore throat settles in and your sinuses start pounding, most people want names.

The good news is, if you wash your hands and try not to touch your face too much when around sick people, you greatly lessen the chances of getting sick and passing along an infection. You can find more on this type of prevention in Chapter 6.

IMMUNITY ALERT

Hand sanitizers are a great way to "wash" your hands on the go. They do not, however, remove particle contaminants as well as scrubbing with good old soap and water.

Dealing with Illness

No matter how strong your immune system is, getting sick is inevitable. What matters is how you deal with this illness. First of all, work hard to not spread the infection to others. Take off of work and keep a distance from enclosed spaces full of people. Wash your hands frequently and cover your mouth when you sneeze. Though usually you want to stay active, at times when you are ill your body needs to channel its energy to fighting the infection, and therefore rest is more worthwhile.

Even more importantly, you can use these infections to your advantage. It is through getting ill that your body progressively builds immunity to more illness. This is predicated upon the idea that your body has a good memory response to the illness so it can better anticipate and fight these infections later in life.

In other words, by handling infections early in life, your body will develop more antibodies—that adaptive immunity—so that later in life as your immune system naturally weakens you will be less susceptible to infections that have an even greater effect on your health and productivity as you get older. In other words, a strong immunity now will contribute to a strong immunity later.

That is not to say you want to go out and get yourself sick to develop greater immunity. Rather, you want to do whatever you can to strengthen your immune system so that your immune memory will be as strong as possible if you do get sick.

If you apply the methods in this book, you can get sick less, have less severe and shorter infections, and live an overall healthier life. First, though, let's take a look at the influence your immune system has on the other systems in your body so you can understand how having weak or strong immunity can impact your overall health.

The Least You Need to Know

- Immunity not only protects against infection, but can also decrease your risk of cancer.
- A diseased immune system can not only be too weak, but also too strong and need to be suppressed, requiring you to boost your natural immunity.
- Early exposure to allergens and other substances determines the degree of your sensitivity to them.
- Taking care of your own immunity also lessens the chance that you'll pass infection along to someone else.

Immunity and Overall Health

In This Chapter

- Inflammation and its effect on your health
- Immunity and your heart health
- How immunity affects your brain
- The organs of the immune system

Your immune system works closely with all the major systems in your body. In some cases, vital organs are actually part of the immune system. In other cases, the immune system has tremendous effect on the well-being of an organ, such as your heart or your brain. Tying all these connections together is the basic immune response of inflammation. Inflammation is the canary in the coal mine—testing for it can show that other problems exist—and when chronic, it can actually cause some problems, too.

This chapter discusses the link between immunity and inflammation, your heart, your brain, and other organs in your immune system.

How Inflammation Affects Your Health

Inflammation is a healthy response of the body to injury, infection, and other stresses. When you sprain your ankle, for example, it becomes painful, red, swollen, and warm to the touch—that's inflammation. Your body produces inflammation so it can begin the healing process in the affected area.

Inflammation doesn't just act on traumatic injury; it also acts on anything that doesn't belong in the body, such as a sliver or other foreign object and the pathogens that cause infection. For example, if you cut yourself, the wound may become infected, causing inflammation. Your immune system uses inflammation to isolate, fight, and eliminate the infection. Inflammation increases blood flow and brings many factors—ranging from nutrients to immunologic factors—to the area to either heal or isolate and eliminate unhealthy tissue.

Injury and infection are not the only causes of inflammation. Damage to tissue will result in inflammation, and damage to the blood vessel walls surrounding the heart—such as in atherosclerosis—will increase inflammation in those walls. Cancer cells are also known to increase inflammation.

While short-term inflammation may be a useful part of the immune response, having increased inflammation over an extended period of time is considered unhealthy.

What Contributes to Inflammation

Many factors contribute to the level of inflammation in your body:

- Allergies or sensitivities
- Autoimmune disease
- Burns
- Some chemicals, such as asbestos, artificial sweeteners, and certain plastics
- Certain foods, including foods high in simple carbohydrates and saturated fat
- Foreign bodies, including dirt and splinters
- Infection
- Injury
- Obesity

- Stress
- Toxins, including pesticides and secondhand smoke

As you can see, inflammation is caused by both factors you cannot control (such as infection, injury, and the environment) and factors you can control (such as diet, obesity, and stress). Some factors, such as injury and infection, are considered acute because they last for a short duration of time. Others, such as autoimmune disease and obesity, are long-term or chronic conditions that can prove destructive to your health.

IMMUNITY ALERT

Alcohol is technically a toxin and, when consumed in excess, can increase inflammation.

Immunity and Other Risks of Inflammation

A clear association has been found between weak overall immunity and higher levels of inflammation. The main theory behind this is that when you have generalized chronic inflammation, more immune factors are being used throughout the body, leaving less available to fight acute infections. It has also been shown that vaccines that boost immunity reduce chronic inflammation (see Chapter 5 for more on vaccines).

Excessive immune reactions can increase inflammation as well. In autoimmune reactions, the immune system is overactive and hurts various organs. Whether from having poor or excessive immunity, a low-level inflammatory or immune reaction that persists throughout the body has destructive effects and can cause damage to blood vessels, tissues, and more.

Chronic inflammation—whether caused by weak or overactive immunity—is associated with various health conditions, including the following:

- Arthritis
- Cancer

- Dementia
- Diabetes
- Heart disease
- Osteoporosis
- Stroke

IMMUNITY ALERT

Heart disease, cancer, and stroke are the three most common fatal diseases in the United States. You can reduce your risk of all three by adopting immune-boosting habits, such as getting proper nutrition, exercising regularly, and managing your stress levels.

How Inflammation Is Measured

Certain types of inflammation can be difficult to observe. Fortunately, your doctor can measure your level of inflammation with a simple blood test. The test looks for various *biomarkers*, like the following, that indicate the type of inflammation you are experiencing.

DEFINITION

Biomarkers are markers of biological process. In the case of inflammation, biomarkers are used to identify the presence and severity of inflammation in your body.

C-reactive protein (CRP) is the primary indicator of inflammation in your body. The higher your CRP level, the greater the amount of inflammation you have. Though a good measure of chronic inflammation, changes in CRP are more sensitive to acute changes in inflammation.

Erythrocyte sedimentation rate (ESR) indicates certain types of arthritis and inflammatory bowel disease, such as Crohn's disease and colitis. It is also an indicator for Hodgkin's disease. ESR is less sensitive than CRP to changes in acute inflammation.

Homocysteine is an amino acid that occurs in the blood. High levels of homocysteine can indicate that your arteries are damaged, leading to atherosclerosis and possibly the formation of blood clots.

Lp-PLA2 travels with "bad" or LDL cholesterol in your blood. High levels of Lp-PLA2 indicate the possibility of atherosclerosis.

Considering that inflammation has been linked to serious health conditions such as heart disease, autoimmune disease, and cancer, this test is well worth your time.

If you are unable to get this test through your own doctor, you may have some alternative options you can turn to, such as WellnessFX (see Appendix B).

How to Reduce Inflammation

Reducing your inflammation levels is an important step in the right direction to ensuring better health. The following are actions you can take to reduce inflammation:

- Manage your stress (see Chapter 8).
- Eat an immune-boosting diet (see Chapter 9).
- Get plenty of exercise (see Chapter 7).
- Avoid foods and chemicals that cause inflammation (see Chapter 9).

All of these interventions will also boost your immunity, which will help further control inflammation. Essentially, certain activities that improve your overall health and immunity will lower your inflammation, which in turn will improve your health further.

IMMUNITY ALERT

Excessive exercise (more than 90 minutes of daily, intense exercise) has been associated with an increase in inflammation.

Knowing Your Heart

Your heart is a vital organ. Together with your blood and blood vessels, your heart is part of your circulatory system. Without your heart to pump life-giving blood through your circulatory system, you would die.

Your heart pumps blood throughout your body via a complex network of veins and arteries. Blood contains red blood cells, white blood cells, platelets, and plasma. Each of these components performs an important function:

- Red blood cells: transport oxygen
- White blood cells: fight infection
- Plasma: transport nutrients and waste products
- Platelets: help blood clot

When your heart functions properly, it pumps about 1,900 gallons of blood each day. That's a lot of blood, and it's all necessary for your health and survival.

Unfortunately, the heart doesn't always function properly. Heart attacks and heart failure are exceedingly common. In fact, heart disease is the most common cause of death and disability in the United States. What scientists are learning is that the immune system plays a critical role in determining heart health.

How Immunity Affects Your Heart

About 71 million people in the United States suffer from cardiovascular disease, mostly caused by *atherosclerosis*. In many of these cases, a strong connection exists between atherosclerosis and chronic inflammation, which is caused by having a chronic suboptimal immune response.

DEFINITION

Atherosclerosis is the buildup of plaque in your blood vessels that obstructs blood and oxygen flow to vital organs. It's also referred to as "hardening of the arteries."

How your immune system responds to atherosclerosis contributes to heart disease. When LDL (bad) cholesterol transports fats and cholesterol to artery walls, it damages and clogs your arteries. Your immune system detects the damage and does its job, showing up to fight the foreign substance (the cholesterol deposit) and repair the damage to the artery wall. Unfortunately, this can prove problematic.

When your immune response kicks in, the artery becomes inflamed, and the immune cells come to fight the foreign substance. As they work away on the damaged artery, they create plaque, which constricts blood flow through the artery. Additional inflammatory responses weaken the cap on top of the plaque until, eventually, the cap bursts and travels to where it might clog a blood vessel.

When the cap on the plaque bursts, your platelets spring into action to form a clot in the problem area. This is exactly what they are supposed to do. Sadly, the result of all these aspects of your body doing its job can be a blocked blood vessel that can't feed your heart enough of the oxygen- and nutrient-rich blood it requires to survive; this dangerous situation can result in a heart attack and possibly death.

Beat Your Risk Factors for Heart Disease

Many risk factors contribute to heart disease. The fewer risk factors you have, the better your chances of preventing heart disease. Fortunately, you can influence the presence of risk factors by changing your lifestyle and, if necessary, taking certain medications.

IMMUNE BOOSTER

Work to eliminate any risk factors for heart disease that are within your influence—lose weight, exercise, eat right, and quit smoking (if you do smoke). The fewer your risk factors, the better your chances of preventing heart disease.

The major risk factors are as follows:

- Family history
- High blood pressure
- High cholesterol (specifically, LDL cholesterol)
- High triglycerides (fats in the blood)
- Obesity
- Sedentary lifestyle
- Smoking

Some of these risk factors are genetic. If you have a family history of heart disease, for example, your best bet is to focus on reducing or eliminating all the other risk factors. If diet and other lifestyle changes alone don't fully lower your blood pressure or LDL cholesterol, you may need to take medications. However, making lifestyle changes should always be the first step.

If your risk factors are genetic, you should at the very least have your blood pressure checked regularly and your triglyceride and cholesterol levels checked annually—more often if you have problematic readings. If your blood pressure is too high, you may need to go on a low-sodium diet. Eliminating sources of bad fats, such as red meat and certain baked goods, can help address any high triglyceride and LDL cholesterol levels you have. You also have the option of taking medications to control your blood pressure and cholesterol levels.

Many people mistakenly believe that having high overall cholesterol is unhealthy. The truth is, you want to have high *good* cholesterol, or HDL cholesterol. You can improve your HDL cholesterol by eating fish and other foods high in good fats, such as omega-3 fatty acids. See Chapter 9 for more on what makes a fat good or bad.

IMMUNE BOOSTER

You can increase your "good" fat intake by eating fish. Many types of fish, such as salmon and tuna, are high in omega-3 fatty acids, which can promote healthy HDL cholesterol levels. If you are unable to eat fish, try taking fish oil supplements.

As for the other risk factors—smoking, obesity, and sedentary lifestyle—you can take charge of your health, changing your lifestyle to diminish or eliminate most of them. If you smoke, quit. If you are obese, change your diet to a heart-healthy, immune-boosting diet and get some exercise. If you are sedentary, start walking a little each day.

Exercise and healthy eating are the cornerstones of a lifestyle that will keep your heart healthy and boost your immunity. Though making these changes takes some work, your immune system will thank you. (We offer more information on how to make these kinds of changes in Part 2.)

Your Immunity and Your Heart

You may be surprised to learn that your immune system plays such a significant role in your cardiovascular health. But it's true—the healthier your immune system, the healthier your heart, and vice versa. These two systems are closely reliant on each other, which can make understanding their relationship a little confusing.

Inflammation, a basic immune response, is the golden thread that connects these two systems. A high level of inflammation can indicate that something may be wrong with your cardiovascular health. It also signifies that your immune system may be in a state of chronic response, which is not good. In this state, your immune system becomes overburdened and is less able to fight off infection and disease.

Because inflammation and heart disease are intimately connected, damage to your blood vessels can cause inflammation, and conversely, inflammation can cause damage to your blood vessels. Therefore, by both lowering your inflammation and improving your heart health, you boost your immunity.

You can't feel inflammation, so how do you know if it's normal or elevated? Luckily, you can find out your inflammation levels simply by having a blood test (see the section "How Inflammation Is Measured," earlier in this chapter). Once you have these test results, you and your doctor can determine the best course of action, which may include further, targeted testing to figure out the cause of the inflammation, some modifications to your lifestyle, or both. Many physicians feel that inflammation testing should be as common as cholesterol testing and be performed on everyone once they enter their 20s and early 30s.

It's also valuable to get your cholesterol and blood pressure tested. Both are major risk factors for cardiovascular disease, which as you know is closely related to your immune health. So what you do to improve your immune system will improve these risk factors as well. (See Chapter 13 for more on testing your cholesterol.)

Beyond tests, you can improve your heart health and also your immunity through diet, exercise, and stress management (see Part 2 for more on these topics).

Your Brain and Immunity

Your brain is command central for everything that happens in your body. If you think it, feel it, taste it, hear it, or see it, your brain makes that happen. Your brain controls your movements—even the ones you are unaware of—and the function of all the systems of your body.

Like your brain, your immune system is also tied to most aspects of your physical health. All of your systems—digestive, respiratory, circulatory, and more—are heavily affected by your immune system. With all that overlap, it's probably unsurprising that your immune system and your brain work pretty closely together.

This is actually great news. By improving your brain health, or your mental health, you can boost your immunity—and the reverse is true, too.

The Brain-Body Connection: Your Mental Health

Your mental health is the single biggest influencer of your stress hormones, most notably cortisol, a potent immune suppressor. This is just one aspect of the brain-body connection that scientists have been studying for many years.

Just as significant as the cause of stress is the way you manage stress. Stress can be short term or chronic in nature. Long-term, negative feelings of anger, sadness, and fear can lead to chronic stress and have a harmful effect on your immune system.

To improve your mental and immune health, you must find the best ways to deal with and eliminate stress. In some cases, that may mean eliminating the cause or changing the way you cope. Easier said than done? Maybe, but with time, you can accomplish it. Check out Chapter 8 for ways you can manage stress.

IMMUNE BOOSTER

The best way you can improve the effect your brain has on your immune system is by decreasing your stress, whether it's through relaxation, deep breathing, or medication.

Stroke

Atherosclerosis doesn't just affect the arteries to the heart; it affects the arteries to the brain, too. Because of this, having atherosclerosis increases your risk of stroke. Stroke occurs when a blood clot or bleeding stops the flow of blood to the brain, similar to how a blockage to the heart can cause a heart attack. A stroke is essentially a "brain attack." Depending on how many brain cells are deprived of blood and for how long, a stroke can cause paralysis or even death. You can have many small strokes or one big one. Like heart disease, stroke is a leading cause of death and disability in the United States.

The following are the warning signs of a stroke:

- Sudden numbness or weakness on one side of the face, arm, and/or leg (symptoms on the face can be on the same or opposite side of the symptoms on the rest of the body)
- Sudden confusion; trouble speaking or understanding

- Sudden trouble seeing in one or both eyes
- Sudden trouble walking; dizziness; a loss of balance or coordination
- Sudden, severe headache with no known cause

If you have a stroke and are less mobile, your immunity will suffer (see Chapter 7 for more detail on how physical activity can affect your immunity). Fortunately, many of the interventions in this book that help your immunity also reduce your risk for atherosclerosis, which in turn can lower your risk of a stroke.

IMMUNITY ALERT

If you suspect that you or another person is having a stroke, call 911 for emergency medical care right away. The sooner a person receives treatment, the greater the chances that permanent damage can be avoided.

Boosting Your Brain Health

As with the heart, what's healthy for the immune system is also healthy for the brain. Chronic inflammation has been linked to many brain conditions, including dementia and Alzheimer's disease. And certainly, chronic inflammation is tied to cardiovascular disease, which can result in heart attack or stroke. So you have everything to gain by investing in the health of your immune system.

The best way to control chronic inflammation is to tame the chronic immune response your body is suffering. In addition, you can use nonmedical and medical interventions to control the atherosclerosis that happens in your brain. First, though, have your CRP and cholesterol levels checked to establish a baseline as a point of comparison for the future. Your doctor may choose to follow up these simple blood tests with other testing, depending on the results.

As with any medicine, you'll do best to meet the traditional treatment halfway. For example, if you take medication to manage your cholesterol, it doesn't make sense to load up on a high-fat diet. That would defeat your best efforts. Make dietary changes and incorporate or increase your exercise to make your solution an integrated one, which will be more effective. In fact, lifestyle interventions should always be your first intervention when it comes to improving your brain health. Unlike prescription medications, these interventions will only have positive side effects and will cost much less (see Parts 2 and 3 for lifestyle changes you can make to boost your immunity and therefore your brain health).

Decreasing the Risk of a Brain Tumor

Many people don't realize the immune system actually helps suppress cancer. Your immune cells identify cancer cells as foreign, and your immune system sets out to destroy them. Most of the time, it works—the cancer is either eradicated or its growth is slowed down. Sometimes, however, a cancer goes undetected or grows too quickly and overwhelms the immune system. When this happens, medical testing and treatment are important. Early detection is vitally important with all cancers.

Among the most common cancers known to be sensitive to the immune system are *lymphomas* of the brain. Studies show an impaired immune system actually increases the risk of this sort of tumor. Therefore, a healthy immune system can actually decrease the risk of a brain tumor.

DEFINITION

Lymphoma is a tumor in a lymph node, as is seen in Hodgkin's and non-Hodgkin's lymphoma.

Prevention is the best medicine, in all cases. But first, you need to know where to start. Have your physician check your CRP levels (see the section "Measuring Inflammation" for more on this test). From there, your doctor will work with you to uncover the source of any chronic inflammation you're suffering. The best news would be that you're carrying no chronic inflammation. But finding out you have a problem isn't bad news—it just means you can get the jump on it.

Either way, you will benefit by taking steps to boost your immunity. Getting good nutrition, exercising regularly, and reducing stress all go a long way toward improving your immune and overall health and reducing inflammation. All of these benefits decrease your brain cancer and general cancer risk.

Organizing Your Vital Organs

Many of your organs serve some sort of immune function, even if that isn't their primary purpose. Most of the following organs are vital, and slight variations in their functioning can affect your immune system. So much of boosting your immunity entails taking care of these organs.

Kidneys

When they function properly, your kidneys filter the bad contents in your blood, similar to your lymphatic system (see Chapter 1). This steady flow of improper substances out of your blood and into your urine decreases your exposure to inappropriate substances. When their functioning is compromised, however, your kidneys may not do a good job of filtering the stuff that should not be in your blood.

Kidneys may also pass too many substances, not reabsorbing and holding onto that which is essential for the immune system. For example, most of the immune system is composed of proteins, including antibodies. One of the first signs of an improperly func-tioning kidney is the wasting of proteins into the urine. By losing protein in the urine, you lose a valuable component of your immune system.

IMMUNE BOOSTER

To help keep your kidneys flowing, try to drink eight 8-ounce glasses of water per day. If you drink diuretics like caffeine or alcohol, take in extra water to prevent dehydration, which can decrease flow to the kidneys.

In addition to testing your urine for protein, your kidney function can be assessed with some simple blood tests. Two substances, blood urea nitrogen (BUN) and creatinine, are filtered by your kidney, and excess amounts of them in the blood can be reflective of the kidney not filtering enough. The difference between the two is that BUN is smaller, so it gets reabsorbed by the body so it will be higher in times of dehydration, when the kidney is reabsorbing excess amounts. By testing these, your doctor or an online service can assess your kidney function and hydration status.

Liver

The liver performs over 300 vital functions in your body, including filtering toxins, producing proteins, making hormones, aiding digestion, manufacturing clotting factors, and much more. Because one of the key functions of the liver is filtering or deactivating toxins, many of the nonfood items you ingest initially go to your liver, including alcohol and medications. These substances irritate the liver and often can damage liver cells. In terms of immunity, the liver produces proteins that are essential for immune function.

Your liver has an amazing ability to heal, but excess irritants can overwhelm the liver's healing mechanisms. Unfortunately, you often don't see signs of liver dysfunction until the liver is 90 percent damaged. And dysfunction of the liver causes decreased immune protein production and therefore decreased antibodies and other proteins essential for optimal immune function.

To maximize the liver's capability to manufacture immune factors, you want to minimize damage to liver cells. Therefore, if you drink, decrease your alcohol consumption, which is highly toxic to the liver. And because medications and over-the-counter drugs such as acetaminophen (Tylenol) can irritate the liver, try to minimize your use of strong prescription medications (though some medications may be unavoidable) and not take higher than the recommended dosages. Finally, if you're overweight, work on bringing your weight down through diet and exercise; excess weight can be damaging to the liver because the fat can get stored there.

Blood tests that check for liver inflammation (aspartate aminotrans-ferase and alanine aminotransferase), functioning through clotting (prothrombin time, partial thromboplastin time, and international normalized ratio), and protein production (albumin, globulin, and total protein) will help you know if your liver is irritated. Consider obtaining these tests through your doctor or alternative health and wellness service.

Lungs

Your lungs improve your overall health and immune system by breathing in oxygen, which, while essential for optimizing many of the body's functions, is also quite toxic to many types of infections. By having good lungs, you maximize oxygenated blood flow to all of your tissues, which improves their overall health and decreases their risk of infection.

Your lungs are exposed to the outside environment, which is why pneumonias in the lung are among the most common infections. To help decrease the amount of these infections, your lungs have their own innate immune system with various immune cells in the lung tissue that identify and attack offenders that are breathed in. They also have certain components, such as little hairs called *cilia*, which repel irritations out of the lungs.

If lung function worsens, such as in pneumonia or excessive inflam-mation in your lungs, you can't take in as much oxygen, which hurts your immunity as well as your overall organ function. The easiest way to optimize lung function is to not smoke (see Chapter 5) and to not breathe in other harmful substances, such as asbestos, coal dust, or silicon. While checking lung function is not as easy as a blood test, your oxygen status will often be checked at a routine doctor visit with a simple instrument called a *pulseoximeter*, which is placed on your finger and can determine the oxygen saturation of your blood using infrared technology.

Bowels

The bowels, or lower digestive tract after the stomach, are perhaps the most interesting organ linked to the immune system. They are chock full of immune tissue, and although this can be harmful in rare instances—such as with autoimmune disease and allergies—in general, this can be very beneficial to the body. The bowels are constantly exposed to various offenders; the lymphoid tissue in the bowels fights them off. Maintaining healthy lymphoid tissue in the bowels, therefore, is essential to your immunity and overall health.

You can actually use this lymphoid tissue to improve your overall immune health by adding healthy bacteria to boost the tissue's functioning. The bowels contain a lot of healthy bacteria that constantly stimulate the lymphoid tissue to promote more immune fighters throughout the body. It has been shown that increasing these healthy bacteria can further boost your immune system. This is the whole concept behind probiotics: by supplementing these bacteria, you increase your whole-body immunity (see Chapter 12 for more on probiotics).

IMMUNITY ALERT

When you take antibiotics, be sure to take a probiotic supplement—either through pills or yogurt—to preserve as much good bacteria as possible.

Spleen

The spleen is actually a part of the immune system. It has a lot of lymphoid tissue and acts as an essential part of the lymphatic system. It's stocked with white blood cells to fight infections and acts as one of the main areas where infections get sequestered and destroyed. Similar to how the lymph nodes swell when there's an infection nearby, your spleen swells when you have certain infections.

The spleen can be removed if necessary, as it's not essential. But those who have had their spleens removed are at increased risk of certain infections, such as pneumonia and sepsis. Because of this, those without spleens are encouraged to get certain vaccines to decrease the risk of these infections (see Chapter 5 for more on vaccines).

The Least You Need to Know

- Have your doctor test you now for chronic or elevated inflammation to establish a baseline. The test, a CRP test, is a simple blood test.
- High LDL cholesterol and an increased immune response cause atherosclerosis, which can result in a heart attack or stroke. So get your cholesterol and CRP levels tested regularly.
- A strong immune system can suppress atypical cancer cells, which can help prevent certain brain and other cancers.
- Boosting your immunity involves taking care of your immune organs—kidneys, liver, lungs, bowel, and spleen.

Giving Your Immune System a Fighting Chance

Part

2

The great thing about immune health is you can take action to improve it and make tremendous gains. This part provides a road map for what you can do to help your immune system operate at peak performance. You find out about the importance of getting vaccines, not just for you and your health, but for the health of all those around you. If you're a parent, this part also gives you information on how breastfeeding and early exposures to potential allergens and sicknesses can boost your child's immunity right up through adulthood.

In this part, you also learn that the best defense is a really great offense. Knowing the best way to wash your hands, the right way to clean, and what to do when you can't avoid exposure to infectious agents all play an important role in keeping your immune system working properly.

Perhaps most important, in this part you get the rundown on the lifestyle changes you can make that will boost your immunity. Getting regular, moderate exercise and practicing stress reduction through relaxation, deep breathing, and meditation are shown to have tangible benefits on your health. Add quitting smoking and limiting drinking to that list, and you're headlong on the right path to optimal immune health.

Your Immunity Toolbox

Chapter

5

In This Chapter

- Building immunity with vaccines
- Boosting childhood immunity
- How your age and your genes influence your immunity
- Bad habits you can break to improve your health

The most effective treatment for any infection is prevention, and the best tool in your arsenal is vaccination. You can support your health—and the health of your children—by getting vaccines and their appropriate boosters. By doing this, you boost immunity both in the present and for your later years, when immunity can often decline.

Other interventions can also increase your immunity as you age, including taking action to increase the genetic expression of immune-boosting factors and doing away with harmful habits.

In this chapter, we look at vaccines in detail and discuss the influence age and genes have on your immunity. We also look at the bad effects smoking and drinking can have on you and what you can do to quit such immune-weakening habits.

Vaccines: The Ultimate Immune Booster

Vaccines are the single most effective way of improving your immunity. Vaccines work via *sensitization* to prevent diseases that could become serious even with treatment.

> **DEFINITION**
>
> **Sensitization** is when an antigen is administered to provoke an immune response. This way, the body has a stronger response the next time it sees the antigen and therefore is able to better deal with the exposure.

Vaccines protect you from disease by mimicking an antigen and provoking a response from your immune system. Once you receive the injection—usually by injection, though some vaccines are administered orally or through inhalation—your immune system learns how to eradicate the germ (or microbe) that attacks it, greatly reducing or eliminating the chance of future infection by that microbe. When your body is able to fight off the infection on its own, you are said to be immune to that infection.

According to *Understanding Vaccines: What They Are, How They Work* (see Appendix B), traditional vaccines contain microbes that have been killed or weakened so they can't cause disease. When these weakened or dead germs enter your body, they elicit an immune response. By provoking a response from your immune system, vaccines train your immune system to fight off the real microbes when it encounters them down the road.

Two types of vaccines are used: live, attenuated vaccines and inactivated vaccines.

Live, attenuated vaccines contain living microbes, which are weakened (attenuated) so they can't cause disease. This type of vaccine is closest to the real thing, so it elicits a strong immune response that can confer lifelong immunity, often with only one or two doses. The downside is that these vaccines can change to a disease-causing state before the vaccine is administered.

Inactivated or *killed vaccines* contain dead microbes. The microbes are killed by using chemicals, heat, or radiation. Unlike live, attenuated vaccines, inactivated vaccines can't change to a disease-causing state. On the flip side, most inactivated vaccines stimulate a weak immune system response when compared with that of live vaccines. So it generally takes several additional doses, or booster shots, to maintain your immunity with this type of vaccine.

No matter the type of vaccine you take, vaccination helps protect entire communities from certain diseases that are passed from person to person and achieve herd immunity. Herd immunity, as you'll recall from Chapter 3, provides protection to people who are unable to receive certain vaccinations by limiting their exposure to the contagious diseases.

IMMUNE BOOSTER

Vaccines are usually administered by injection, but some vaccines can be administered orally or through inhalation.

Diseases to Vaccinate Against

According to *Understanding Vaccines: What They Are, How They Work*, in the nineteenth and early twentieth centuries, certain illnesses were a subject of extreme worry. In the United States alone, hundreds of thousands of people, mostly children, were infected with these illnesses each year, and without vaccines or effective treatment for these illnesses, tens of thousands of people died each year. Today, the following diseases are all but forgotten largely because of vaccines.

Diphtheria is a bacterial infection with complications that include heart swelling and failure. Diphtheria can be prevented by the DT and Tdap vaccines.

Hepatitis A is a viral infection in the liver that can result in acute liver failure. Hepatitis A can be prevented by the HepA vaccine.

Hepatitis B is a viral infection of the liver that can lead to chronic liver failure and liver cancer. Hepatitis B can be prevented by the HepB vaccine.

Human papillomavirus (HPV) is a viral infection that causes genital warts and cervical cancer. HPV can be prevented by the HPV vaccine.

Influenza, commonly known as the flu, is a viral infection that can cause mild to severe illness and is sometimes deadly. Your risk for influenza can be reduced by a yearly flu vaccine.

Measles is viral infection that can cause rash, cough, and conjunctivitis (pinkeye) and lead to pneumonia, brain damage, seizures, or death. Measles can be prevented by the MMR vaccine.

Meningococcal disease is a bacterial infection that causes bacterial meningitis—an infection around the brain and spinal cord—in children, as well as blood infections. About 1 in 10 people who get the disease dies from it. Lasting effects may occur, including loss of limbs, deafness, neurological disorders, seizures, or strokes. Meningococcal disease can be prevented by the MCV4 vaccine.

Mumps is a viral infection characterized by fever, headaches, and painful swelling of the salivary glands under the jaw. It can lead to meningitis, inflammation of testicles or ovaries, and deafness. Mumps can be prevented by the MMR vaccine.

Pertussis, commonly known as *whooping cough,* is a bacterial infection marked by severe cough and, in infants, apnea (a pause in breathing). It can result in pneumonia or death. Pertussis can be prevented by the Tdap vaccine.

Pneumococcal disease can cause blood infection, meningitis, and death. Pneumococcal disease can be prevented by the PCV13 vaccine.

Polio is a viral infection that can cause paralysis and death. Polio can be prevented by the IPV vaccine.

Rubella, also known as the German measles, is a viral infection that's mild in children and young adults but can cause miscarriage, stillbirth, premature delivery, and birth defects in pregnant women. Rubella can be prevented by the MMR vaccine.

Tetanus, also known as lockjaw, is a bacterial infection that involves stiffness in the neck and abdominal muscles and difficulty swallowing. Tetanus bacteria are found in soil and spread through exposure to cuts in the skin. Tetanus can be prevented by the Tdap vaccine.

Varicella, commonly known as *chickenpox*, is a viral infection with symptoms that include itchy rash, tiredness, headache, and fever. Varicella can be prevented by the varicella vaccine.

Zoster, commonly known as shingles, is a viral infection caused by the same virus that causes chickenpox. The virus lies dormant in a person's system after a chickenpox infection and can resurface as a painful rash later in life. Your risk for zoster can be reduced by the zoster vaccine.

IMMUNE BOOSTER

Review your vaccine status with your doctor. If you are missing any, make sure to get them and find out whether there's a booster schedule with them.

Risks of Vaccination

Prior to vaccines, many more cases existed of pneumonia, meningitis, and various previously deadly infections. Vaccines have greatly reduced many of these once-fatal diseases. The benefit of getting the vaccines—and the risk of not getting them—is substantial. You are far more likely to contract a deadly disease that a vaccine could have prevented than you are to have a severe allergic reaction by getting the vaccine. However, even with all the evidence and history of information showing how vaccines improve the immunity of individuals and communities, some people feel the risks of being vaccinated or having their children vaccinated outweigh the benefits.

The typical side effects of a vaccine—including soreness at the injection site and an assortment of other minor symptoms—are due to the immune reaction it provokes. The common side effects of the flu shot, for example, are hoarseness, itchy eyes, cough, fever, aches, headache, itching, and fatigue.

In the extremely rare instances where severe side effects occur, an allergy to the vaccine is typically the culprit. If you're allergic to eggs, for example, you may not be able to get a flu shot, because it's made using egg protein. Other vaccines may cause different types of reactions and allergies, so it's important to report these allergies to physicians in the future.

In recent years, an erroneous link has been made between vaccines and autism. Studies don't bear out this connection, and it has been shown that children who do not receive vaccines are much more at risk for deadly infections. It is for this reason the American Academy of Pediatrics, the World Health Organization, and the Institute of Medicine say there is no identifiable relationship between the two.

IMMUNE BOOSTER

You can look up the side effects—mild, moderate, and severe—of all vaccinations at cdc.gov/vaccines.

Childhood Vaccines

Pediatricians do an excellent job of making sure children's vaccines are up to date. This schedule, based on guidelines by the Centers for Disease Control and Prevention (see Appendix B), has been developed and revised over many years to create the optimal immune protection for children and also minimizes the number of times children need to go their doctors to receive injections. The following table summarizes the infant and childhood vaccine schedules and the various diseases each vaccine protects against.

Immunizations for Babies

Disease	Vaccine	Recommended Age
Diphtheria, pertussis (whooping cough), tetanus	DTaP	2, 4, 6, and 15 months
Hepatitis A	HepA	12 months

Disease	Vaccine	Recommended Age
Hepatitis B	HepB	At birth, between 1 and 2 months, and between 6 and 18 months
Hib (*Haemophilus influenza* type b)	Hib	1, 4, 6, and 12 months
Influenza (flu)	Influenza	6 months through 18 years
Measles, mumps, rubella	MMR	Between 12 and 15 months
Pneumococcus	PCV	2 months, 4 months, 6 months, and between 12 and 15 months
Polio	IPV	2 months, 4 months, and between 6 and 18 months
Tetanus	DTaP (also protects against diphtheria and pertussis)	2, 4, 6, and between 15 and 18 months
Varicella (chickenpox)	Varicella	12 months

Immunizations for Children

Disease	Vaccine	Recommended Age
Diphtheria, pertussis (whooping cough), tetanus	Tdap	11 and 12 years
Human papillomavirus (HPV)	HPV	11 and 12 years
Influenza	Influenza	Yearly
Meningococcal conjugate	MCV4	11 and 12 years, with a booster at 16 years

Adult Vaccination Boosters

Though most vaccines are administered in childhood to offer the greatest protection, sometimes vaccines need to be administered into adulthood. This could be because certain vaccines require boosters to stay effective, specific diseases are more prevalent in adulthood, or some viruses mutate and require more up-to-date vaccines to offer continued protection. The following table summarizes the current adulthood vaccination schedule, based on guidelines by the Centers for Disease Control and Prevention (see Appendix B). You will notice far more range in when adults can receive certain vaccines than children.

IMMUNE BOOSTER

Keeping a vaccine card will help you track your previous immunizations and your future immunization schedule.

Immunizations for Adults

Disease	Vaccine	Recommended Age
Human papillomavirus (HPV)	HPV	Between 19 and 26 years for women (3 doses); between 12 and 21 for men (3 doses)
Influenza (flu)	Influenza	Every year
Measles, mumps, rubella	MMR	Between 19 and 50 years (1 or 2 doses)
Pneumococcus (pneumonia)	PCV	65 years
Shingles	Zoster	60 years
Tetanus, diphtheria, pertussis (whooping cough)	Td/Tdap	Get Tdap once and then a booster every 10 years
Varicella (chickenpox)	Varicella	Between 19 and 65+ years (2 doses)

Helping Children Build Immunity

When children are first born, they do not have a fully developed immune system and are at a much higher risk for infections, some of which can be deadly. That's why when a baby has a fever, far more tests are performed to look for serious bacterial infections than if it were an older child. Young infants—especially infants born prematurely—are at much higher risk for pneumonia, meningitis, and urine infections. Young girls, because of their shorter urethras, are at a much higher risk for urine infections during their first couple years of life.

Babies' immunity starts to develop rapidly, though, partly with the aid of vaccines. Risks for infection greatly decrease at 1 month, 3 months, 6 months, and 2 years, similar times to when many vaccines are administered. Vaccines are also given at these intervals so the immune system can deliver the appropriate response.

Another aid to babies' immunity during this dangerous time is the antibodies they get through their mother from breastfeeding, which is discussed next.

The Benefits of Breastfeeding

Breastfeeding provides babies with antibodies and white blood cells that help them fight infection until their immune systems are able to do so on their own. The American Academy of Pediatrics recommends that mothers breastfeed their babies for the first year. If this isn't possible, try breastfeeding for the first two to three months when the neonates in their immune systems are the weakest. However, breastfeeding for the entire first year is still ideal.

IMMUNE BOOSTER

Colostrum, the premilk produced in the breast during the first few days after birth, is especially dense with disease-fighting antibodies.

Sometimes it's not possible to breastfeed a baby. Certain health conditions or medications may preclude you from breastfeeding, or sometimes, the baby or your body just won't cooperate. That's okay.

If you are unable to breastfeed your baby, consult with your pediatrician to come up with a nutrition plan that is beneficial to developing your baby's immunity. Baby formula has been improved very much over the years, and although breastfeeding is more advantageous, your baby can grow up to be quite healthy even if bottle fed.

Early Exposure

A lot of immunity, as well as allergies, is influenced by exposures during childhood. Certain food or environmental exposures too early in life can cause a negative sensitization that manifests as allergic reactions later. On the other hand, too little environmental exposure can make the body not get used to certain exposures, which can manifest later as allergic reactions or lack of immunity to such exposures. In other words, following general pediatric guidelines, which are well researched, about when to start various foods affects your child's health during childhood and throughout adulthood.

Furthermore, it's probably not beneficial to keep children away from all infectious exposures when they are 2 to 10 years old (as opposed to neonatal age, when they are very high risk) because it's with these exposures that people develop their immunity that persists through adulthood. While parents may hate it when their kids get sick, some of that is beneficial for forming adult immunity. Again, children less than a year old are a special case, as they are much higher risk and should be kept from being exposed to various infections if possible.

Nutrition and Rest

Kids who eat a diet that includes plenty of fruits and vegetables are more likely to be healthier and less likely to suffer diseases (such as cancer and heart disease) during adulthood (see Chapter 11 for immune-boosting foods and Chapters 14 and 15 for immune-strengthening recipes).

IMMUNE BOOSTER

The key to getting children to enjoy vegetables is to introduce them to different types when they are young. Try to get your child to eat five servings of fruits and vegetables every day.

And as with adults, when children don't get proper sleep, certain antigen- and cancer-fighting immune cells aren't produced in great enough amounts. This makes children more prone to illness and puts them at greater risk for cancer over the long term.

The following are the recommended daily sleep times for children of various ages, according to the Center for Holistic Pediatric Education and Research at Children's Hospital in Boston:

- Newborn: up to 18 hours per day
- Toddlers: 12 to 13 hours per day
- Preschoolers: 10 hours per day

Take into account the quality of your child's sleep, too. Naptime at daycare is far less restful than an hour earlier to bed at home.

Antibiotics only when Necessary

Most childhood illnesses—colds, flu, the "stomach bug"—are caused by viruses, which cannot be treated with antibiotics. Your doctor will (or should) prescribe antibiotics only when the illness is caused by bacteria, as these are the only infections that respond to antibiotics.

Overusing antibiotics opens the door to antibiotic-resistant bacteria. Infections caused by these bacteria are much more difficult to treat because most antibiotics don't work against them, and the infections can be aggressive. The most well-known of these infections is MRSA, which can be very difficult to cure and is a highly serious infection that you don't want your child (or you!) to get (see Chapter 2 for more information on MRSA).

IMMUNITY ALERT

Antibiotics promote antibiotic resistance and kill healthy bacteria. For this reason, many pediatricians choose to offer a "delayed prescription," where a prescription is written but only started if the infection is still worsening after several days.

Don't be afraid to ask your pediatrician whether antibiotics are actually necessary to treat your child's illness or whether the illness can be observed. Some doctors may be tempted to prescribe the medicine because they think you want your children to have one, but often the child can be observed to see if the illness persists or gets worse, as most viruses improve within a few days.

Your Age and Genes

You can't change your age or your genes—or can you? Much research has been done in these areas, and the findings have been encouraging. You may not be able to change your genes, per se, but you can make the most of what you have—which will also affect how well you age.

Age and Immunity

As you get older, your body's genes tend to make less protein, in the form of both immune-type proteins and antibodies. This increases the chance of various infections, especially pneumonia and urinary tract infections (since these areas are exposed to the outside world).

It also means that older people may not manifest many of the typical symptoms of infections, like fever, because of their weaker immunity, so symptoms may just be weakness or confusion. By the time older people are expressing fevers, infections may be fairly advanced. Therefore, older people, like infants, should have a lower threshold for seeking hospital care.

IMMUNITY ALERT

Your chronological age may differ from physiological age, which is a bigger determinant of your immune health. By adopting immunity-boosting habits, such as getting proper nutrition and reducing stress, you can lower your physiological age and boost your immunity.

It's especially important for older people to practice many of the interventions in this book as early as possible and get annual vaccines and boosters (like the flu vaccine) because they are a high-risk population.

Genes Vary in Expression

The mechanisms of various genetic expressions aren't well understood, but we at least know you aren't just stuck with your genes—you can make the most of what you have.

Genes heavily influence people's immunity, starting with genetic immune deficiencies. But even if people don't have an immune deficiency, some have better immunity genes than others. Some people's genes prompt the creation of more immune proteins and immune cells. So children of people "who never get sick" are more likely to have the same level of immunity.

It is believed that certain activities, including physical activity and stress reduction, can also influence expression of these genes. Part of the mechanism of your immune system is that certain genes get expressed to produce more immune proteins. This can happen in injury and infections and is part of the evolutionary process to survive infections.

The genetic expression of immune proteins can also be increased or not decreased through a decrease in the production of immune-suppressing stress hormones, such as cortisol. The following section covers some ways you can make this happen.

Adjusting Your Gene Expression

Cortisol is an immune-suppressing stress hormone (see Chapter 9 for more on cortisol). If you can moderate the amount of cortisol in your body, you can adjust your gene expression to help your immunity. The basic prescription is to practice balance and moderation, with a few tricks to get the gears moving in the right direction.

The following are some ways you can reduce your cortisol levels:

- Manage your stress levels (see Chapter 8).
- Exercise, which naturally drives a lot of the immune proteins (see Chapter 7).
- Get enough rest at night. (Yes, you really do need eight hours of sleep every night!)

- Get good nutrition and eat properly (see Chapter 9).
- Consume probiotics, which stimulate lymphoid genes to produce more immune factors (see Chapter 12).

IMMUNE BOOSTER

Eating healthy foods and getting regular exercise will encourage your genes to make more immune proteins and decrease your risk of infections.

Harmful Habits

Certain chronic habits are known to be harmful to your immunity and your general health. Alcohol and smoking in particular are very destructive to your immune system, and chronic use can significantly increase your risk of infections.

The single most important factor in determining how successful you'll be in kicking a destructive habit—such as smoking or drinking—is the desire to do it. The pro of leaving the behavior behind must outweigh, in your mind, any advantage of retaining the habit. If you truly want to boost your immunity, you should want to kick these habits. Ask yourself, "Which do I want to do more: boost my immunity, or damage my health through smoking or drinking?"

Quit Smoking

Smoking has many effects on the immune system, ranging from paralyzing the cilia in your lungs that repel infectious organisms, to causing inflammation, to generally weakening all aspects of your immune system.

Quitting smoking is a matter of weighing the benefits of quitting against the perceived benefits of smoking. The easiest way to do this is to look at the facts. The following are some of the 7,000 chemicals that cigarette smoke contains:

Tar is the term for all the various particles contained in cigarette smoke. Tar is sticky and brown and coats your lung tissue. It contains carcinogens that promote tumor growth.

Carbon monoxide is a gas that's fatal in large doses. It's the same stuff that comes out of the exhaust on your car or off charcoal from your barbecue grill. When you smoke, you inhale carbon monoxide instead of oxygen, which means that less oxygen reaches your cells, including those in your brain and your heart.

Hydrogen cyanide damages the cilia (tiny hairs) inside your lungs. The cilia are what keeps your lungs clean, so when they are damaged, the toxic chemicals of cigarette smoke stay in your lungs.

Free radicals are chemicals that can damage the heart and blood vessels. They combine with cholesterol to create plaque on artery walls, which can cause heart disease, circulatory disease, and stroke.

Arsenic, cadmium, and *lead,* and other cancer-causing metals, as well as *various radioactive compounds,* can also be found in cigarette smoke.

Remember, that's just a sampling of the 7,000 chemicals other than nicotine in cigarette (tobacco) smoke. The effects of smoking on your respiratory and circulatory system are devastating, even life-threatening. The following lists how smoking affects your immune system:

- Smoking is a general immunosuppressant, which can make you both more susceptible to infections and have a harder time recovering from those infections.

- Smoking paralyzes the cilia, or small hairs in lungs that usually repel infections, making you more prone to respiratory infections—including bronchitis, pneumonia, and influenza—and slowing your recovery time.

- Smoking reduces the amount of antioxidants in your blood and promotes immune-damaging free radicals. (Free radicals are discussed further in Chapter 10.)

These are just some of the effects of smoking on the immune system. Smoking and its effects on your heart, lungs, and even your reproductive and dental health are also well documented.

Chewing gum and nicotine patches are well-known aids to help you quit smoking gradually. Medications, such as Chantix, are also available if you want to quit but are struggling. In fact, so many options are available it can be difficult to know where to begin. If you'd like more information about quitting smoking, including access to a counselor and other tools you can use to help you quit, check out smokefree.gov.

Stop Drinking

Alcohol can inhibit the production of immune and other cells by affecting DNA synthesis. In addition, if alcohol begins to damage you liver, the production of proteins such as antibodies decreases.

Unlike smoking, where any amount of smoking is destructive to your immune and overall health, drinking has been shown to have some benefits (mainly cardiovascular) when consumed in moderation. The trick is understanding the meaning of "moderation."

As a general rule of thumb, one drink on occasion is fine. Three or more—especially if done every day or almost every day—is way too much.

Measurements matter. One drink equals:

- 12 ounces of beer
- 5 ounces of wine
- 1 ounce of liquor

IMMUNE BOOSTER

To get a feel for how much alcohol is in a 5-ounce glass of wine, fill a measuring cup with 5 ounces of water and pour it in a wine glass. You can do the same with 1 ounce of liquid to visualize that, too. Twelve ounces of beer, of course, is just a can of beer.

Drinking too much alcohol harms your immune system in many
ways:

- Overdrinking prevents your body from absorbing
  nutrients, causing nutritional deficiencies that inhibit the
  production of immune cells and proteins.
- Alcohol can impair the ability of immune cells (white cells)
  to kill antigens.
- Alcohol in high doses suppresses the ability of immune
  cells (white cells) to multiply.
- Alcohol in high doses inhibits the action of immune cells
  (killer white cells) on cancer cells.

The more alcohol you consume, the worse the effects on your
immune system. In general, if you feel intoxicated, your immune
system feels some pain as does your body.

If you want to decrease your alcohol consumption but are struggling,
addiction counseling and support groups, such as Alcoholics Anony-
mous (aa.org), can help. Inpatient and outpatient detox programs are
also available to help you quit alcohol.

The Least You Need to Know

- Vaccines are the number-one way to build your immunity.
- Building children's immunity is an investment in their future
  health.
- You can't change your genes or your age, but you can affect
  how your genes are expressed.
- Quit smoking and stop drinking to improve your immune
  and overall health.

Infection Prevention and Minimization

In This Chapter

- How to wash your hands
- Keeping your environment disinfected
- Knowing when to stay home—and what to do when you can't

To ward off infection and thereby maintain a healthy immune system, you should first actively avoid being exposed. Unfortunately, as you learned in previous chapters, living in a completely sterile environment is not only impractical, but potentially harmful to your immunity as well.

In times when you can't avoid exposure, it's important to practice good hygiene to minimize the risk. Good hygiene begins with hand washing and sanitizing the surfaces in your home and extends to preventing the spread of infection among entire groups of people.

This chapter discusses prevention tips to keep your immunity high, as well as ways you can minimize your exposure to infection at home and in the world at large.

Awash in Hand Washing

The most common way that infections spread is through direct contact between an infected person and an uninfected person.

The uninfected person gets the pleasure of catching the infection and possibly passing it along to another unlucky soul, and so on. Fortunately, this cycle of spreading infection doesn't always have to continue—it can stop at you.

Consider how most infections spread:

- An infected person sneezes on, coughs on, or kisses someone who isn't infected.
- An infected person coughs into his hand before shaking hands with someone. The newly exposed person then touches her eyes, nose, or mouth.
- A person touches a surface—such as a toilet handle, sink faucet, or doorknob—where bacteria, viruses, and other antigens have survived.

What all of these methods of transmission have in common is that hand washing—and common sense and courtesy—can play a huge role in reducing the spread of infection.

Washing your hands, done at the right times and in the right way, is the single most effective way to prevent disease transmission and eliminate exposure to a majority of infections.

How to Wash Your Hands

Most people don't wash their hands long enough and in all the essential places. When you wash your hands, really suds up the soap and wash for at least 30 seconds. Be sure to get between your fingers, in the web spaces, and under your nails.

As an alternative, you can use hand sanitizer. Make sure your hands get good and wet with the hand-sanitizing gel and rub it in until your hands are dry.

IMMUNE BOOSTER

A great trick to make sure you're washing your hands long enough is to hum or sing the "Happy Birthday" tune in your head two or three times while you wash.

When to Wash Your Hands

Knowing *when* you wash your hands is just as important as knowing *how* to wash them. Your nose, mouth, and eyes, as well as open cuts, are the entryways to your body that can be infected due to direct contact. Washing your hands at appropriate times—before you eat, after you handle dirty objects, and certain other times—will help keep those entryways safe and you healthy.

According to the Mayo Clinic (see Appendix B), you should always wash your hands before and/or after certain activities, as illustrated in the following table.

	Before	After
Putting in or taking out contacts	X	
Using the bathroom		X
Changing a diaper		X
Touching an animal or anything related to it, such as toys, leashes, or waste		X
Using garden or household cleaners and chemicals		X
Handling garbage or anything that could be contaminated, such as cleaning cloths or soiled shoes		X
Preparing or eating food	X	X
Medical care, such as treating wounds, giving medicine, or taking care of someone who's sick or injured	X	X

In general, you want to get in the habit of washing your hands routinely throughout the day, as you never know if the surfaces you touch are contaminated. For example, money is known to contain various germs. By getting into the habit of keeping your hands clean, you can minimize your exposure to various infections, no matter what you come into contact with.

It is especially important for kids to clean their hands—children are notorious for spreading infections, so if you have kids, make sure they wash their hands properly. Extra care is also required among or around people with weaker immunity, including newborns (or neonates), the elderly, and immune-compromised people. If you're around one of these higher-risk groups, you should wash your hands often.

Picking a Hand Cleanser

Washing your hands with any type of cleanser will eliminate most germs. Even washing with plain tap water—with no soap at all—can wash away bacteria. Your best option is to wash with soap and water, especially when you have particulate matter—or, more scientifically put, "stuff"—on your hands.

Depending on what's on your hands, you may choose to use anti-bacterial soap instead of regular soap. For example, if you have been handling raw meat or cleaning cat litter, you may want to use the stronger soap. For general cleaning, however, go for the plain soap, because overusing antibacterial soap diminishes its effectiveness fighting against bacteria.

When soap and water are not available or convenient, another option for cleaning your hands is to use hand sanitizers (usually a gel made from alcohol and a few other ingredients) or hand wipes. Look for a hand sanitizer that's at least 60 percent alcohol, and when possible, opt for the gel rather than the wipes, which don't get your hands as wet with the sanitizing agent.

IMMUNITY ALERT

Note that hand sanitizers aren't as effective as good old soap and water. They will eliminate most flu viruses, but they score poorly when used to clean bacteria or cold virus. While using them is better than using nothing, don't rely on hand sanitizers as a primary cleaning method.

Keeping Your Environment Disinfected

The next most effective way to avoid infection is to keep your environment clean. This sort of hygiene involves cleaning the surfaces in your home, at work, and in your car. Any place or thing you touch with your hands or put in your mouth—such as dinnerware, writing or eating utensils, and toothbrushes—must be sanitized to reduce the risk of infection.

Of course, the surfaces that tend to collect bacteria and viruses are the surfaces you touch the most. Your hands are the most contaminated "surface" in the house—think of all the things your hands come in contact with throughout the course of a day and in between washings. That's a lot of germs! So washing your hands combined with sanitizing the surfaces in your home are the most sensible steps you can take to lessen your risk of infection.

How Infections Spread from Surfaces

Many people think they can only catch a cold or the flu by shaking hands or sharing a drink with an infected person. The truth is, when a sick person sneezes or coughs into her hand or blows her nose into a tissue and doesn't wash her hands before touching a surface, the surface becomes infected. You can then catch the person's cold or flu, or other infection, by touching the surface with your hand and then touching your eyes, nose, or mouth. The flu virus can live on certain surfaces for 72 hours, so you can imagine how unsanitary the surfaces can be in public places such as the mall, restaurants, or public transit stations.

Surfaces can also be infected in other ways that don't require touch. Toothbrushes kept in the bathroom are listed as one of the most infected surfaces in a typical home. Think about this: every time you flush the toilet, germs from the toilet spray 6 to 10 feet in the air. If your toothbrush is exposed on the side of the sink near the toilet, how gross is that? This is why you should sterilize your toothbrush every week or, preferably, store it in an enclosed area away from the toilet.

IMMUNE BOOSTER

To prevent the spread of infection, make sure your toothbrush dries completely between uses, especially when you're sick. And be sure to disinfect it once a week, using very hot water and an antibacterial soap, and let it dry completely.

With surfaces, the solution is two pronged. First, you need to keep the surfaces sanitized in places you can clean (such as your home, office, car, and so on) and be mindful about touching surfaces in public places. Second, you must practice good hygiene. When you touch a surface that may be infected, wash your hands, and whatever you do, don't touch your eyes, mouth, or nose.

The Most Common Places for Bacteria and Viruses

Germs love moisture, which is why sink drains, your toothbrush, and kitchen sponges are among their favorite places to flourish. Anywhere you touch with your hands—whether it's your phone, the TV remote control, or your computer keyboard—is a breeding ground for bacterial and viral infections. In addition, anything you use to eat or drink is a hotspot for infection. Anywhere that has organic matter has germs—that's just the way of it. What you may find surprising, though, is just how extensive the list of affected surfaces is.

Kitchen:

- Countertops
- Cutting boards
- Dishes waiting to be washed in the sink, on the counter, or in the dishwasher
- Dishwasher drain
- Garbage bin
- Garbage disposal
- Kitchen surfaces
- Refrigerator
- Sink

- Sink drains
- Sponges and washcloths

Bathroom:

- Bathtub (especially whirlpool bathtubs)
- Faucets
- Grout
- Shower head
- Shower liner
- Sink drains
- Toilet
- Toilet handle
- Toothbrushes
- Towels and washcloths

Bedroom:

- Blankets and sheets
- Mattress
- Pillows
- Shoes

Living room:

- Children's toys
- Furniture
- TV remote control

Home office:

- Computer keyboard and mouse
- Phone
- Touchscreens

Laundry room:

- Dirty laundry
- Washing machine (behind seal, drain, wet clothes)

All rooms:

- Door knobs
- Floors
- Light switches
- Tabletops

All of these must be disinfected regularly. These surfaces also get contaminated at work and other facilities, so make sure to try and maintain hygiene when out.

Washing your hands before and after touching hotspots, like the kitchen sink and computer keyboard, will go a long way to helping you stay healthy.

IMMUNITY ALERT

The most infected surface in a house is usually children's toys, and the most prevalent germ is the flu virus.

How to Stay Sanitary

After reading the list in the preceding section, you may think staying sanitary is an exhausting task, but it's not. All you really need are some basic tools and good hygiene habits. Because surfaces can be stubborn to clean, look for antibacterial and antiviral cleaners. And don't worry; surface cleaners don't have the same risk of resistant bacteria occurring as antibacterial hand soaps.

While cleaning products may not seem to be related to immunity, remember the single most effective way you can decrease your risk of infection is maintaining a hygienic environment. To help maintain that environment, the following are the basic types of cleaning products you need:

- Bleach or a bleach-based product—for kitchen and bath surfaces
- Ammonia or an ammonia-based product—for glass and fixtures
- Antibacterial liquid soap—for finished wood and a catch-all for anything that's not bleach or ammonia friendly
- Antibacterial floor wash—for the type of flooring in your home

While bleach and ammonia are the most potent cleansers, they aren't suitable for many surfaces. Therefore, use other antibacterial cleansers for surfaces that can't handle those products.

IMMUNE BOOSTER

For an easy way to clean light switches and cabinet handles, use a disinfecting wipe. You may also find bleach or other disinfecting wipes helpful for wiping down your computer keyboard or TV remote control.

Surrounding Yourself in Health

Practicing good social hygiene helps you minimize your exposure to infection and makes you less likely to pass along infection to others.

This is especially important during the winter months, when people spend more time indoors in close contact with one another. It is a myth that it is just the cold that "gives you a cold"; in fact, it is due to this proximity that more infections are spread in the winter, as opposed to the cold weather itself.

The more people who practice good social hygiene, the healthier everyone can be.

Avoid Sick People

When it comes to supporting your immunity by reducing infections, the best defense is a good offense: avoid sick people.

That sounds easy enough, but you really can't avoid all people, and you can't trust sick people to isolate themselves. Furthermore, you may not even know which people are sick. In fact, they may not know that they're sick. Infections tend to be most contagious very early in an illness, and it's only later, after people realize they are fully sick, that the contagiousness of the infection rapidly decreases.

If you see people who are visibly sick, though, take note of it and take immediate precautions. Give them some distance so they don't cough or sneeze on you. And if you notice people sneezing and coughing, give them space. Stay out of the trajectory of the spread of germs, as many droplets can travel several feet after a sneeze or cough.

Avoid shaking their hands or hugging and kissing hello, and if you cannot avoid it, immediately cleanse your hands after. You may not be able to avoid contact altogether, but you can still minimize your exposure.

IMMUNE BOOSTER

One of your authors is an emergency physician who sees many sick people every day and has to touch them to examine them. By simply washing hands before and after every patient and doing other immune-boosting techniques, rarely does the author ever get sick.

Don't Be the Spreader

You actually have two opportunities to stop the infection cycle: you can avoid contracting the infection, or you can avoid spreading the infection. Part of having good social hygiene is knowing when you need to hold back so you can avoid infecting other people when you're sick.

You may think, *Why do I care about giving infections to other people?* For two reasons: First, by supporting other people's health, you boost the immunity of those around you and therefore decrease the risk they later develop an infection that's passed along to you. Second, you should always follow the golden rule: treat others as you wish to be treated. If everyone cared about passing on infections, it would decrease your risk of receiving an infection. Therefore, by setting the example of not being the spreader, you lessen the chance that someone may spread an infection to you.

If you're coughing or sneezing uncontrollably, you should stay home from work and social engagements. Staying home from work in particular can be a difficult decision—deadlines loom, and the pressure to be present is palpable. Some professions are more forgiving of sick time than others. Can you work from home? Can you take sick time? Will people at the office really want you there if they know you're sick? Know what's best for your health and your career.

Productivity can also increase when a culture of responsible hygiene exists, because the number of people who are out sick decreases when infection isn't passed around the office. In other words, overall work productivity actually increases when people stay home when they're ill. If everyone does their part, a culture of responsible hygiene can exist.

 IMMUNITY ALERT

When the H1N1 (swine) flu was prevalent, people were encouraged to wear face masks to protect themselves against infection. In actuality, the people who should have worn the masks are the people who had the infection. Masks offer little protection to the uninfected.

Protect Yourself from Airborne Illness

You know the time—flu season. The stomach flu is going around, and everyone has a cold. Sometimes, none of that matters. You have to go to work; you have to hit the grocery store; you can't get out of the holiday festivities because you're the one hosting the party. In addition, sometimes you can't avoid trains, planes, and automobiles that put you in close contact with many other people, some of whom may be ill.

You can become infected by direct contact (as covered previously in this chapter), but you can also become infected by germs that are spread in the air, through sneezing or coughing. These germs spread through water droplets or on dust particles you inhale. Like any virus, the flu can spread this way, as can the common cold. Since droplets can travel several feet, you want to keep your distance from anyone visibly and repeatedly coughing or sneezing.

Fortunately, people know more today about the spread of germs and some ways they can help diminish its effect. The days of coughing and sneezing into your hands have past. Instead, you should cough into the crook of your elbow. This decreases contamination of your hands, which reduces the spread of infection by direct contact. Because your sneeze and cough are covered by your elbow, the spread of airborne germs is also reduced.

Another method that works to reduce the threat of infection is to practice hand awareness. When you practice hand awareness, you divide tasks between your hands and stay aware of which hand you use for which tasks. So, for example, you can use your left hand to touch your eyes, nose, or mouth and your right hand to shake hands with people and experience any other exposures. Combined with frequent hand washing, hand awareness can make a difference in your level of exposure.

Of course, the best awareness is knowing when you should wash your hands, whether that's due to your hands coming into contact with contaminated surfaces or people or being sick yourself. By repeatedly cleansing your hands when you are ill or around others who are ill, you will spread your germs to fewer surfaces and protect other people from getting sick.

The Least You Need to Know

- Wash your hands with soap and water for 30 seconds before you eat, after you handle dirty objects, and other times you are exposed to germs.
- Disinfect the surfaces in your home to avoid infection.
- Stay healthy, and keep others around you healthy, by practicing good social hygiene.

Getting an Immune-Boosting Workout

In This Chapter

- The benefits of exercise and physical activity
- Setting goals and getting active
- Exercise hazards to avoid

Along with good nutrition, exercise is the cornerstone of a healthy, immune-boosting lifestyle. When you exercise regularly, you feel better physically and emotionally. This chapter offers some specifics about the benefit of exercise, especially as it relates to the immune system, as well as the tools you need to create a fitness plan and stick to it. But there can be disadvantages to exercise, so this chapter also discusses overexercise and other potential hazards that can have damaging effects on your body and immune system.

Why You Should Exercise

Exercise helps you feel better and have more energy. Done regularly, physical activity may even help you live longer. If those reasons are not enough, consider the Mayo Clinic's seven main benefits of exercise (see Appendix B):

1. **Exercise helps you control your weight.** Exercising can help you maintain or lose weight, as well as prevent you from gaining unwanted pounds.

2. **Exercise combats diseases and other health problems.** Exercise improves your immune health and helps you ward off heart and cardiovascular disease, certain types of cancer, osteoporosis, and diabetes, to name just a few.

3. **Exercise enhances your mood.** Physical activity stimulates the production of endorphins and other brain chemicals that boost your mood and help you feel happier and more relaxed.

4. **Exercise is a great energy booster.** Exercise helps your heart and lungs work more efficiently, which gives you more energy throughout the day—even when you aren't exercising.

5. **Exercise can help you sleep better.** Regular exercise can help you fall asleep faster at night and sleep more deeply so you feel more rested the next day.

6. **Exercise can improve your sex life.** The physical benefits of regular exercise—increased energy and an improved physical appearance—can lead to a more satisfying sex life. Women who exercise experience enhanced arousal for sexual activity, and men are less likely to suffer from erectile dysfunction.

7. **Exercise is fun.** Exercise and physical activity, once you get into it, can be fun. And you don't have to go it alone—join in group activities or competitive sports to add enjoyment to your workouts.

IMMUNE BOOSTER

Underlying the many benefits of exercise is that exercising is good for your self-esteem. When you are active, you feel better physically *and* mentally.

Compare that with the risks of being sedentary—increased "bad" (LDL) cholesterol and decreased "good" (HDL) cholesterol and a higher risk of heart disease, high blood pressure, cancer, osteoporosis, type 2 diabetes, and depression—and you can see why exercise is important to your health.

In addition, if you spend most of your time sitting or not moving, you tend to be less productive. The illnesses associated with sitting lead to lost productivity, too.

So why not exercise? You have everything to gain by increasing your physical activity—and much to lose by staying sedentary.

The Direct Immune Response to Exercise

Active people have been shown to have much better immune systems than their inactive counterparts. Medical scientists have several theories as to how exercise increases immunity:

- By boosting your heart rate, exercise increases the volume of blood that circulates through your lymphatic system. The lymphatic system serves as the drainage and cleaning system for your blood, so by increasing the flow of blood through it, you improve the health and immunity of your blood.

- Regular exercise helps moderate the amount of cortisol in your blood over the long term, reducing chronic inflammation and boosting your immunity.

- Exercising may flush out cancer-causing cells by increasing the output of sweat and urine from your body.

- Your body temperature increases while you work out. For your body, this is kind of like having a fever, which is the body's natural way to fight off bacterial infection.

- Staying active may help flush bacteria from the lungs, decreasing your chance of catching a cold or the flu.

IMMUNITY ALERT

Researchers from the University of North Carolina in Chapel Hill found that reproductive-age or postmenopausal women who exercised between 10 and 19 hours each week had a 30 percent lower risk of breast cancer.

The Indirect Immune Benefits of Exercise

Indirect benefits to your immunity are actions you take that improve other aspects of your health, which then support your immunity as well. The list of indirect immune benefits of exercise is extensive. Here are just some of the benefits you stand to gain:

- Combats heart disease
- Lowers your blood pressure
- Boosts your HDL cholesterol
- Decreases your triglycerides (which is important for heart health)
- Decreases your risk of cardiovascular diseases
- Prevents stroke
- Manages metabolic syndrome
- Prevents or manages type 2 diabetes
- Manages or wards off depression
- Prevents certain types of cancer
- Manages or even prevents certain types of arthritis
- Improves your balance (which is important as you age)

Remember, improving overall health improves your immune health. So gaining these indirect benefits of exercise helps boost your immunity just as much as gaining the direct benefits that improve immune health.

The Fitness-Mood-Health Connection

Exercising regularly improves your overall sense of well-being.

For one thing, exercise is a natural antidepressant—it simply makes you feel better about yourself. When you exercise regularly, you are more energetic and healthier. Moderate exercise also dissipates stress by working the stress hormones, including cortisol, out of your system. And, when done regularly, exercise creates endorphins, the hormones that give you a "runner's high"—that great feeling of near-elation.

Because of the brain-body connection, those good feelings you gain from regular exercise also improve your immune system. As stress decreases and endorphins increase, your immunity gets a naturally positive boost (see Chapter 8 for more on stress and its effects on the immune system).

Once you feel the fitness, mood, and health benefits you get from exercising, you'll naturally want to continue. So lace up your shoes and get your heart pumping!

Pump Up the Immune

So you're ready to get started. You have your sneakers, your workout clothes, your bike helmet, your free weights, and your resistance bands. Now what?

Relax—this is the fun part! First things first: you need to create a fitness plan (which you can find more information on in the next section). Because this book is about boosting your immunity—which means getting your blood moving and creating a lifelong plan of healthy living—the fitness plan focuses on performance goals, not weigh-in goals. However, if you want to lose weight, the plan can also support that goal.

After you create the plan, you'll learn some exercises that support good immune health and where you can do them. And to keep you on track, we give you some ideas for how to exercise even while on the job, so you can put your health and fitness first.

 IMMUNE BOOSTER

If you are exercising to lose weight, create a plan that has you losing 1 to 2 pounds per week—anything faster is unhealthy and unsustainable. Remember, fitness is a lifestyle choice, not a destination.

Creating a Fitness Plan

The tough part with any fitness plan is staying motivated. Part of staying motivated is knowing yourself well enough to know what will personally motivate you, but there are some things that have been shown to work for most people.

The first thing you should do is set small, achievable goals and keep track of your progress in an activity log. The journey to meeting these goals should challenge you, but you don't want to set a goal that's so far reaching or aggressive that you lack a sense of forward motion and give up before you really start.

For example, you decide you're going to work out on a treadmill to get started. Most treadmills have variable speed and incline settings and can track your time, distance, and heart rate. You may say, "I'm going to work out for 20 minutes three times a week." But that's not really specific enough, and it also may not be interesting enough to keep you going over the long term. You need a sense of forward motion or progress.

Instead, give yourself a more specific, short-term goal, like, "I'm going to walk 1½ miles in 20 minutes." Log your progress as you go, on a sheet of paper, a wall calendar, a spreadsheet program, or your favorite fitness app on your smartphone. Then, when you achieve your goal, up the ante on yourself. Maybe bump up the speed or play with the incline. Have you been monitoring your heart rate? If you've been at the low end of your aerobic level, push to a higher level (but not too high—you'll read more on the dangers of that in the next section). For example, you can modify your goal to "I'm going to walk 2 miles in 30 minutes at an incline setting of 2." With that more aggressive goal, you then need to create steps toward meeting that goal. So maybe for the first week, you raise the incline for 5 minutes of your workout, followed by 10 minutes for the second week.

Remember, your fitness journey is ongoing. You should constantly be setting new goals and committing yourself to them. Be realistic, challenge yourself, and above all, have fun!

IMMUNE BOOSTER

If you have a smartphone, you may find it fun to track your fitness progress on one of the many fitness apps. See Appendix B for some of our favorite options.

What Is the Best Form of Exercise?

Now that you've figured out a fitness plan, it's time to decide what exercises will best help you boost your immunity. There are three basic types of exercise:

- Strength training (weights)
- Aerobic (cardio)
- Flexibility (stretching)

Strength training increases fast-twitch power glycolytic muscle (responsible for quickness and strength), which supports release of growth hormone, an immune enhancer (the opposite of cortisol). Strength-training exercises should be rotated to include a day of rest after a certain body part is exercised. For example, if you work out your arms on Monday, give your arms a rest and work out your legs on Tuesday. By Wednesday, you can return to your arms. Core muscles—those in your torso—are an exception to this rule and can be worked out every day. The following are some different strength-training exercises:

- Free weights
- Weight machines
- Resistance bands
- Other resistance training (such as push-ups and other exercises in which you use your own body weight as resistance)

Aerobic exercises support slow-twitch oxidative endurance muscle (responsible for long-term endurance) and lymphatic flow. There are many different types of aerobic exercise. You should try to get at least three days of aerobic exercise for at least 30 minutes a session. More is better—up to a point (more on that later in this chapter). The following are some of the more popular aerobic exercises:

- Walking
- Running
- Cycling (biking)

- Swimming
- Working out on various training equipment, (such as a treadmill, elliptical, stationary bicycle, recumbent bicycle, or rowing machine)
- Aerobic dance classes (such as low-impact and high-impact classes, step classes, Jazzercise, and Zumba)

While flexibility is often overlooked as an important part of any exercise routine, it is essential if you want to develop better balance and stay limber as you age. In addition to standard stretching, you can try the following to increase your flexibility:

- Yoga
- Dance
- Any of the popular martial arts disciplines (such as karate or tae kwon do)

In addition, many competitive and team sports offer a lot of the same aerobic and strength-training benefits as personal exercising:

- Baseball or softball
- Basketball
- Football and tag football
- Golf
- Hockey
- Lacrosse
- Racquetball
- Soccer
- Tennis

When you choose an exercise activity, choose one that's fun and enjoyable to further motivate your progress. If you're a group person, join a team or take a class. If you're a solo competitor, break out your own personal scorecard and chart your progress on an activity log.

Whatever you do, be active. It's the best thing you can do for your health and therefore your immune health.

> **IMMUNE BOOSTER**
>
> Many individuals find greater motivation and effort in engaging in competitive exercise. The game distracts from the exertion, and after the match they find they have had a much better workout than just doing noncompetitive fitness activities.

Choosing a Location

When you're just starting out, you need to consider where you'll exercise. Do you wish to exercise at home or at a gym? Whatever your choice, it should be a place that's comfortable, affordable, and easily accessible.

First, consider your comfort level working out with other people. Do you like having the camaraderie and added motivation of seeing others working out close by, or do you feel better when you're exercising alone at home? If you feel comfortable working out with others, you may want to try a trial gym membership to see how you like it. Different gyms have different "personalities," and one may be a better fit for you than another.

Next, consider the expense. If you decide to work out at home, the cost doesn't have to be very expensive—with some free weights (dumbbells and ankle weights), resistance bands, a mat, and a good pair of sneakers, you can be well on your way. Having a treadmill or other piece of cardio equipment can also be useful; if you can't afford it, though, you may fare just fine walking or jogging outside. For rainy days, you can pick up a DVD or one of the many cable channels that show exercise classes throughout the day. If you're joining a gym, you'll have to pay a monthly fee. Some gyms run specials at certain times throughout the year, so pay attention to see what the going rate is. Also find out the gym's cancellation policy. If you don't like the gym for some reason (maybe it doesn't have equipment you like), you should be able to cancel your membership easily with no penalty.

Finally, consider accessibility. Obviously, working out at home is ideal if you want to exercise at a moment's notice. However, working out at a gym requires more attention to this issue. If the gym is 20 minutes away, you've set yourself up an extra obstacle to getting your workout in—a 20-minute ride. So look for something convenient that's either close to home or close to work.

And if you want to get away from home or your gym and add some interest to your usual exercise program, the Adult Education or Parks and Recreation Department, the YMCA, or another local gym may offer classes that you can take once or twice a week. Maybe Zumba twice a week mixed in with at-home strength training and bicycling outside is just the thing for you. You can always try new things, so have fun.

IMMUNE BOOSTER

Remember to keep a fitness log to help you stay on track with your exercise regimen. Record your weight and the type and amount of cardio and strength training you complete each day. Some people find taking motivational photos of themselves every month or so is helpful, too.

Incorporating Physical Activity into Your Day

Some jobs, such as retail or restaurant work, require you to be quite active during the day. You're on your feet carrying heavy objects and managing customers for hours on end. Other jobs, however, have you sitting at a desk much of the day, which is a passport to sedentary living. If you have a desk job, don't lose hope—you can incorporate some physical activity into your day, too.

Ask about getting a stand-up desk for your office. These desks have an adjustable height that can be raised just a little higher than countertop height, which allows you to stand while you work, burning more calories and exercising your legs. You may find that working this way is actually easier on your back, too (unless you have a specific back injury or condition that makes it less comfortable).

You also can stand on a stabilizing board or sit on a stability (balance) ball to work your core stabilizer muscles throughout the day. When you're using the stability ball as a seat, your body is constantly realigning to keep its balance, so you actually burn more calories while sitting.

And don't underestimate the value of a brief walk. Even a brief, two-minute walk every hour helps refresh your body and mind and rev your metabolism. Some people even take "walking lunches" or a 20-minute trek around the office park or city followed by a quick lunch at their desk. Not only can this refresh you—you'll feel as if it's a new day when you return to your desk—it dissipates the cortisol that has built up in your system while you were working away at your desk.

The idea is to get moving any way you can. Active people have been shown on average to live a few years longer than sedentary people. Their quality of life is better—they are healthier, more productive, and happier—so those extra years are a welcome addition to their time. You can start your journey to a healthier and immune-boosting lifestyle, and potentially a longer life, by including exercise at your workplace.

IMMUNE BOOSTER

Give yourself a complete lifestyle makeover. Don't just increase your activity; make it a hobby. Try subscribing to a fitness magazine or online newsletter to help you stay motivated.

Too Much of a Good Thing?

As wonderful for you as exercise is, overexercising is destructive to your immune health and therefore your overall health. When you overexercise to the point of overtraining, your body is breaking down more than building up. The following sections look at the problems that come with overtraining and offer some insight into how to know when you've crossed the threshold.

The Problems of Overtraining

A major mediator to your body's breakdown from overtraining is cortisol, which suppresses the immune system (see Chapter 9). Higher levels of cortisol are seen after an hour and a half of moderate exercise and increase during prolonged, intensive exercise. This is especially the case if you have not eaten during the few hours prior to exercise, because your body has to create more energy on its own. This stress on the body can lead to chronic inflammation and can increase your risk of infection.

Long periods of exercise, such as long-distance running or intense bodybuilding workouts, can actually decrease the number of white blood cells circulating through the body and increase the presence of cortisol and other stress-related hormones, which further suppress the immune system. For the most part, the immune weakening that appears shortly after long-distance workouts seems to be temporary and is followed by an enhanced immune response. In other words, long endurance training, if not overly taxing to the body, still supports the immune system even though it suppresses during and shortly after exercise.

But it's not always easy to know when you're overdoing it, especially when you've worked hard to keep a forward progression going in your performance.

How to Know when Enough Is Enough

People are most likely to overdo it when training for an event, such as a 5k or a marathon. However, it's possible to overexercise just out of pure zeal, too. The following are some signs that you may need to slow down, based on information from *U.S. News & World Report:*

- **Decreased performance.** Is it suddenly harder to keep pace with yourself, or are you finding your feet feel "heavy" under you?
- **Mood changes for the worse.** The same stress hormones released when you're mentally burdened or overworked at your job are also released when your body is physically overtaxed.

- **Persistent muscle soreness.** If you're still sore days after you exercise, you need to rest until you recover and proceed at a more moderate pace when you return. That soreness is telling you your muscles are still recovering from the micro-tears of exertion, and doing strenuous exercise again will retard recovery.

- **Elevated heart rate.** When you exercise regularly, your heart rate will go down as you get in better shape. If you overdo it, however, your heart rate may actually increase because of the strain of overexercising.

- **Mental and physical fatigue.** If you're working out at a high level for you or for long durations (say, an hour and a half per workout), you may experience fatigue.

- **Insomnia.** Regular exercise helps normalize sleep patterns. Overexercising, however, can disrupt sleep patterns by causing excess release of stimulating adrenaline that provides energy for exercise, but can create difficulty sleeping.

- **Loss of muscle mass.** If you're gaining fat and losing weight overall, you're losing muscle. This means your body is overproducing cortisol (the immune-busting hormone) and harm is being done to your immune system and therefore your body.

- **Weakened immune system.** If you let things get out of control, your immune system will begin to really suffer. You can experience inflammation, infection, and even injury.

IMMUNITY ALERT

If you suddenly start experiencing insomnia, try stepping your exercise regimen back a bit. Also, be sure that you're not working out too close to bedtime.

Other Immune Risks of Exercise

It's not just overtraining that can potentially harm your immunity; environment and equipment are also potential hazards to your health.

In nature, for example, if you train outdoors in cold weather, you'll be exposed to elements such as cold air and wet weather. These can increase the stress on the body, increasing cortisol and weakening the immune system. In addition, the dry air can create cracks in the nasal mucosa, where viruses can more easily penetrate. If you exercise in this kind of weather, try wearing tight undergarments and a face mask to stay warm and protect you from the elements.

When it comes to equipment, make sure to adequately clean any clothes, shoes, or other equipment you use. Moisture from sweat helps support the growth of bacteria and viruses, and by maintaining dry, clean clothes and equipment, you can help prevent the spread of infections. This is not just applicable to your clothes and personal equipment, but also the equipment you use at other facilities. When working out with gym machines, keep in mind they're touched by lots of people who are sweating and don't necessarily clean the machines between each use, making them a source of infection. Be sure to wipe them down with a disinfectant wipe or spray and paper towel before and after each use. This both protects you from infections and is courteous to other members of the gym.

The Least You Need to Know

- Exercise benefits your immune health and therefore your overall health.
- Set achievable fitness goals and keep a journal or activity log to record your progress.
- When you choose a place to exercise—whether at home, outside, or at a gym—be sure to choose a place that's comfortable, affordable, and easily accessible.
- Avoid overexercising and any equipment and environmental hazards that could weaken your immunity.

The Only Stress Is Stress Itself

In This Chapter

- Recognizing your stress
- Structured relaxation that benefits your immunity
- Deep breathing to improve your health
- Meditation that calms your mind and your body

Together with moderate exercise and a healthful diet, stress management is an important marker in the health of your immune system.

Relaxation that keeps your stress levels low reduces cortisol production, which facilitates good immune health. It also makes your immune system operate more efficiently—all the time spent struggling against cortisol instead can be spent doing what it's built to do: fight infection and detect and eradicate abnormal cells.

In this chapter, you will learn how to recognize and deal with stress in order to improve your immune health.

Coming to Terms with Stress

Your immune system may seem far removed from discussing the nature of stress, but it's not. The connection between a reduction in stress and your overall and immune health has been proven in many studies. But how does stress work, and how can you deal with it?

The Nature of Stress

Your body's stress response is designed to help you power through whatever situation is placing stress on your system. It speeds your heart rate and pushes blood to your muscles so you can engage or get away from whatever is perceived to be a threat. A whole host of physiological responses occur, including increased lung capacity to ensure more oxygenation of your blood and the release of cortisol so food sources and even body tissue can be converted readily to energy. In a sense, you can say that this is a fear response. The body perceives danger, and it prepares to flee or go into battle—a fight-or-flight response.

When you experience stress over the long term—or experience a stress response even when you don't know why you are stressed—all these responses and chemicals in your bloodstream, particularly cortisol, can have a damaging effect on the immune system. You can get sick with infection more easily and have other health problems.

So clearly, reducing stress is a healthy thing to do. Along those lines, the first step to reducing stress is to understand what is causing it.

IMMUNE BOOSTER

When you experience stress during a crisis—such as the death of a loved one, a job loss, or a sudden move to a new home—you may find it helpful to enlist a professional to support you through the grieving or other emotional processes. If you don't know where to start, consider a grief support website, such as griefshare.org.

Many people don't recognize the types of stress they face. The most common types of stressors are the ones you face on a day-to-day basis.

Workplace stress comes from the demands of a job. Most people work more than they historically did, and although the work may be easier (if it's a desk job, for example), it generally requires longer hours and more days, with progressively more and more to do. Because this work setup has become commonplace, many people accept this as a part of life and simply endure, not recognizing what this is doing to their body's critical functions.

Financial stress is as common today as ever. You live in a consumer society. In general, people spend and consume just as much or more than their income. Most households are in the red, with debt exceeding savings. This also ties in to work stress, because the unstable job market makes many people live in fear of losing their jobs and therefore their source of income.

Home stress comes from the day-to-day running of the household. People balance work with managing children, a home, and the rest of their lives. They also put a lot of activities on our kids, which increases their own demands.

Sleep deprivation happens when people don't get the proper type and amount of rest at night. Our ancestors didn't wake up with alarm clocks—rather, they slept until their bodies were rested. Today, people live at a high activity level, balancing career, family, and personal development against taking care of basic needs, such as the need to get proper rest.

IMMUNITY ALERT

Many people compensate for sleep deprivation with caffeine, which raises cortisol levels and creates a stress response. Get rest and avoid caffeine as much as possible to support your immunity.

How Stress Damages Your Body

Times have changed, but people's bodies have stayed more or less the same. When our ancestors came face to face with a wild animal, their bodies would undergo chemical and physiological changes to prepare them to confront the threat or run away from the beast. As mentioned earlier, this is the fight-or-flight response, and you can still experience it today. You don't necessarily encounter life-threatening situations when you experience it, however; you can experience this stress response for far less grave reasons. The stress response may be helpful in the short term, but it can be very unhealthy in the long term. If you don't teach yourself how to relax, you can have chronically high stress levels.

When you experience the fight-or-flight response, your body produces cortisol to raise your blood sugar for more energy. If you'll remember (and as you'll read more about in Chapter 9), cortisol is also an immune suppressor that can have many other harmful health effects. And if you have chronic stress, the increase in cortisol levels suppresses your immune system and raises your blood sugar, putting you at higher risk of diabetes, heart disease, stroke, and more.

Other things occur within your body as you feel stress, too, such as a rise in blood pressure to increase blood flow to your organs. If your stress becomes chronic and your blood pressure is continually high, you're at a higher risk for heart attack and stroke.

Unfortunately, most of the stressors you deal with today (as described in the preceding section) are chronic stresses and not the acute stresses people evolved to handle.

Fortunately, you can manage and even reduce your stress by using relaxation techniques and getting regular exercise (see Chapter 7).

IMMUNITY ALERT

As the brain-body connection has become better understood, many scientists feel that mental stress is now as great if not a greater risk factor for many diseases, including heart disease, ulcers, and even autoimmune disease and dementia.

Coping with Stress

Now that you know how the body's stress response works and how to identify what causes your stress, you can learn to cope. Start by eliminating as many of the stressors as makes sense. For those stressors you can't eliminate, such as cleaning the house or paying bills, incorporate some stress-management habits into your day to help diminish their effect on your immune health.

You may have many stressors: the mortgage, your job, the kids, "getting it all done." You may not be sleeping well because of the stress, which adds more stress on your body, creating a vicious cycle. So what can you do?

First, be honest with yourself. The one thing that all these stressors have in common is you. How do you process the world around you? Do you set limits for yourself so as not to overtax your time and energy level? How good are you at putting yourself first?

If you can put self-care at the top of your list, you will get the payoff with great dividends. Not only will you feel better, you will be healthier. When you put yourself first, you can make healthier choices. For example, if you start each day with exercise, you energize yourself naturally, which means you don't require caffeine and other energy inducers that function by increasing immune-suppressing cortisol. Exercise also decreases the stress response your body has to various stressors.

You might also choose to make lifestyle decisions that decrease your stress. For example, if you don't buy as much and alternatively save and invest, you can have more financial security should you ever face potential money problems, such as job loss. This would give you a greater feeling of autonomy in your occupation, knowing you can better handle financial stressors. Consuming less means less to manage, such as a smaller home with a lower mortgage, a less fancy car, and so on. When you make these choices, you can worry less about your stuff and your finances. In addition, another benefit of consuming less and saving more is you can invest to earn interest, meaning income would be augmented as well. Although this may all seem pretty removed from the immune system, by making these sorts of life decisions and reducing chronic stress, you improve not only your immune system but also many other important aspects of your health.

For those stressors that you can't remove through lifestyle practices and exercise, there are other things you can do to cope, such as relaxation, deep breathing, and meditation. These methods are covered throughout the rest of this chapter.

Relaxation and Your Immunity

Relaxation has been well studied and is shown to have numerous benefits both to your overall health and your immune health.

Practicing relaxation can improve your cardiovascular health, enhance your body's ability to fight cancer, and increase your mental sharpness. With all these benefits, the question of "Why practice relaxation?" quickly falls away, leaving "How can I practice relaxation?"

The Benefits of Relaxation

When you have a full plate of work and personal responsibilities, it's more important than ever to keep on top of practicing relaxation techniques. These are the times when you stand to benefit the most from relaxation, and they are also the times when it's easiest to neglect practicing it.

The following are the benefits of relaxation on your health, as identified by the Mayo Clinic:

- Slows your heart rate
- Lowers your blood pressure
- Slows your breathing rate
- Increases blood flow to your muscles
- Reduces muscle tension and chronic pain
- Improves your concentration
- Reduces anger and frustration
- Boosts your confidence so you can handle problems

In order for you to benefit fully, use the relaxation techniques discussed next in conjunction with the coping methods discussed earlier.

IMMUNE BOOSTER

In addition to the many physiological and immune benefits, relaxation has been shown to improve our mental acuity and energy, which can make you more successful and efficient at the tasks that stress you.

Easy Ways to Relax Quickly

Relaxation is actually a pretty simple concept. The important thing to understand about relaxation is that a little can go a long way. Just by taking a few seconds to do some sort of relaxation—such as pausing to look out your window or taking a moment to enjoy a cup of tea—you can benefit significantly physiologically.

The following are just a few easy ways you can enjoy a moment or two of relaxation during your day. The possibilities are near limitless, as what one person finds relaxation may not be appealing to you, and vice versa:

- Take a few deep breaths.
- Stretch—you can stand or sit to do it.
- Listen to your favorite slow song and align your breathing to the beat.
- Take in the view—look out the window, out the door, or even at a picture on your desk.
- Close your eyes and picture yourself relaxed.
- Drink hot tea. Try chamomile or black tea, which have been proven to reduce cortisol levels.
- Step away from a stressful situation for a few minutes; you'll return refreshed and better able to deal with its challenges.
- Experiment with positive thinking. Instead of imagining the worst possible outcome, ask yourself, "What's the best outcome that could happen?"
- Take a few moments to smile or laugh. Maybe you have a favorite radio program or some music that makes you feel light.

These techniques represent just a smattering of the ways you may find to relax throughout your day. Just know that being aware of your need to relax and then taking steps to relax pays big dividends in your overall and immune health. You're worth it!

Long-Term Stress Reduction Methods

Although you stand to benefit either way, longer practices of relaxation are even more beneficial than short ones. You have time to relax, once you know how to do it. It will become as natural as reaching for a midday cup of coffee (which is counterproductive to relaxation).

The following are just a few ideas for how you can incorporate long-term stress reduction methods into your day:

- Eat a nutritious diet (see Part 3).

- Get moderate exercise (see Chapter 7). However, remember that overexercising can compromise immune function.

- Use deep-breathing techniques (described later in this chapter).

- Try meditation (described later in this chapter).

- Listen to your favorite music or something brand new that appeals to you. Listen to the entire album, front to back.

- Experiment with scents. Place some nearby and rest your body. Many people find the essential oil of lavender to provide a soothing scent. Lavender-scented bath salts are also popular.

- Spend some time outside. Do some gardening or light yard work—even shoveling snow can be relaxing if you're not in a hurry. Or go on a nature walk to clear your thoughts.

- Spend some time alone or with friends. Know whether you need companionship or isolation to relax.

- If you have pets, spend some time with them. Slowly petting cats has been proven to reduce stress.

- If you have children, have a family game night. Nothing takes down your stress level faster than a rousing round of *Candy Land*.

Relaxation is important to maintaining good health. The main takeaway here is that making time for relaxation is not an insurmountable problem. Put your needs first—even if you can grab only a few minutes—and you'll benefit physically and emotionally from your effort.

IMMUNE BOOSTER

When you slow down your breathing, your heart rate naturally slows and the level of cortisol in your body lowers, which boosts your immune system. While you focus on your breath, immerse your mind in something not stressful. Sometimes that means clearing your mind for a bit—and that's fine, too. The idea here is to enjoy yourself.

Reducing Stress Through Deep Breathing

Deep breathing can help induce relaxation and reduce stress, which can have many positive effects on your health. Deep breaths promote blood flow and increase your oxygen intake, both of which offer more oxygen-rich blood to your lungs. Deep breathing also promotes the flow of blood through the lymphatic system, which is a tremendous boon to your immunity (see Chapter 1). Even a few seconds of deep breathing benefits your health.

How Deep Breathing Works

When you breathe deeply, your diaphragm fully extends and contracts, "massaging" your internal organs and making you feel immediately refreshed. After a few deep breaths, the tension in your torso, shoulders, and neck begins to release. Your blood pressure will even drop several points after a few slow breaths—just another benefit of minding your breath.

IMMUNITY ALERT

If you are deep breathing and you feel tingling in your hands or lips, stop the exercise to recover your breath—these are signs of hyperventilation. To avoid this problem, take slower, more controlled breaths.

The deep breaths that calm your body also slow the production of cortisol and other chemicals that are problematic for the immune system. When you perform deep breathing and other relaxation techniques, your cortisol lowers, decreasing its suppression of immune function.

When you breathe deeply, you promote blood flow and increase your oxygen intake, both of which offer more oxygen-rich blood to your lungs. Oxygen-rich blood provides more energy and has more immune-fighting power for your organs and tissues—in fact, oxygen is known to be quite toxic for many infections. Tissues that are oxygen rich are much more able to fight infection.

Deep breathing also stimulates your lung hair fibers, or cilia, and the immune tissue in your lungs to better fight and repel infections. Finally, deep breathing promotes lymphatic flow, which helps cleanse the blood of toxins and antigens. Deep breathing truly is a cleansing process.

How to Deep Breathe

Deep breathing is not so difficult to do, once you get the hang of it. First, assess your current way of breathing. Place one hand on your chest and the other on your belly. When you breathe, which hand moves the most? If you are like most people, the hand on your chest moves the most, meaning you're "chest breathing." You want to work on breathing from your diaphragm so the hand on your belly moves more than the hand on your chest. Some people call this "belly breathing," but it's actually deep breathing.

Now that you know which way you breathe—and have, if necessary, adjusted your breath—you can work on deepening your breathing using slower and more controlled breaths. When you breathe for this exercise, breathe in through your nose and out through your mouth. Count to 10 as you inhale, and then count to 10 again as you exhale. Try to keep your breath steady; it should be one smooth motion where you can inhale or exhale all the way through the last two or three seconds of the count.

IMMUNE BOOSTER

Have you heard the phrase "breathe in blue, breathe out red"? When you draw your long breath, picture the air you are breathing as a liquid, colored blue, that's cool and energizing. Then, when you release your breath, exhale slowly and deliberately, picturing warm, red liquid. This visualization provides tremendous relaxation benefit. Try it!

Using Meditation to Quiet Your Mind

Meditation is a mind-body exercise that has been used for hundreds of years to produce tranquility and a quiet mind. During meditation, you become aware of all the stray thoughts that crowd out your concentration. You then recognize these thoughts and return your focus to whatever the subject of your concentration is—in this case, your breath—to produce a calm and relaxed state. Meditation has been shown to significantly reduce the stress response and, like relaxation and deep breathing, can be done for various durations and in almost any location.

You can explore many different kinds of meditation:

Concentration meditation is the foundation of all other forms of meditation. It concerns bringing your attention into firm focus on an object or activity.

Creative meditation cultivates strength of character by acting as if the character traits you want to have already exist within you.

Heart-centered meditation helps deepen empathy and forgiveness and teaches you to live in gentler ways.

Mindfulness meditation is the form of meditation detailed later in this section because of its ease of use and many health benefits. When you practice mindfulness meditation techniques, you turn your attention to whatever comes into your consciousness. The purpose of mindfulness meditation is to develop a sense of wonder and to see yourself as one part of an interrelated world.

Reflective meditation involves focusing on a theme, question, or other topic. When your mind wanders from that topic, you become aware of it and return your focus to it again.

The Benefits of Meditation

Meditation has been shown to reduce stress in those who meditate regularly, although some short-term benefit is evident after even just one session. The focus on breathing is important; by focusing on your breathing, you become more aware of your body and the emotions you feel. Practicing mindfulness meditation can be a productive way to stay balanced and keep your stress levels in check.

IMMUNE BOOSTER

You may consider taking a meditation class, especially when you are just starting out, in order to learn proper technique and focus. You can even find instructors who do one-on-one instruction.

Mindfulness meditation has been shown to have the following distinct health benefits:

- Improved immune function, including increased antibody creation
- Lowered blood pressure, both during the meditation session and, with regular practice, overall
- Improved cognitive function, including improved ability to concentrate and better memory retention

Mindfulness meditation is the easiest one to begin with (see the preceding section for other types you can explore), so the next section gives you a brief introduction for how to meditate using the mindfulness technique.

How to Meditate

The thing with meditation is that, the harder you to try to do it, the harder it becomes. You have to get out of your own way and let your focus take over. The easiest way to do that is to focus on your breathing.

Think about how time stands still or flies by when you're deeply absorbed in a task, such as reading a book, painting a room, or weeding your garden. When you become deeply focused on the task, your brain quiets down and you reach a state of calm, or flow. This is the state you want to reach when you meditate.

When you meditate, find a comfortable, quiet place to sit or lie down. Close your eyes, and rather than think in terms of clearing your mind, think in terms of focusing on one thing—your breath—very intently. Focus on the rhythm of your breathing, which should be deep and evenpaced. As your mind drifts, be aware of the thoughts that are interrupting your focus and then set them aside as you bring your awareness back to your breath.

The more you practice meditation and focus your complete attention on tasks during your day, the more you will improve your ability to concentrate. This is very healthy for your brain and also benefits your overall health and, of course, your immune system.

IMMUNE BOOSTER

If you have a smartphone, you may find one of the many meditation apps useful. Some have voice-guided meditation or just ambient music. Just pop in your earphones and Zen out for a bit!

The Least You Need to Know

- Address the causes of your stress and use coping skills to manage the stressors you can't eliminate.
- Taking time to relax helps moderate your cortisol levels, which controls inflammation and boosts your immunity.
- Deep breathing slows your heart rate, enabling your body to relax more fully.
- Meditation can benefit your immune function, lower your blood pressure, and improve your concentration and memory.

Immune-Boosting Foods, Vitamins, and Supplements

Part
3

Your immunity is only as good as the food you eat. You can do everything in this book, but if you don't fill up on healthy fuel, you'll see a greatly reduced benefit from what you could have seen had you also adjusted your diet. The highest benefit comes from practicing the whole plan.

This part separates the good from the bad and the misleading when it comes to food. You find out how to distinguish a "good" carb from a "bad" carb and the best type of protein and fats to eat. Preservatives and additives are addressed, as is the way you eat, including how often you eat and how the size of your meals matters.

This part also lays out the facts on vitamins and minerals, explaining which ones provide the most benefit to your immune health and how they do so. You find out about immunity superfoods (yes, they're out there) and which are the best of the best for boosting your immunity as well.

Finally, this part provides information on how you can supplement your immunity with probiotics, herbal supplements, and some DIY remedies. Not all supplements are created equal, so this part helps you find the best for your immune-health needs.

Eating an Immune-Boosting Diet

In This Chapter

- Food and your immunity
- How consuming high-quality carbohydrates, protein, and fats helps boost your immunity
- Preservatives and additives that cause inflammation
- How the way you eat affects your immune health

The secret to a successful immune-boosting diet is balance and moderation. Whether you need to monitor your fat intake, regulate your carbohydrates, or moderate the frequency and size of your meals, balance and moderation are the keys to a healthy eating plan.

Of course, food is one component of a varied lifestyle plan that includes exercise and stress management. You also can assist your body with vitamin and mineral supplements. While all of these interventions and substances are covered throughout this book, this chapter focuses on your basic food.

How Food Affects Immunity

The main substance of the food you eat falls into one of three categories: carbohydrates, protein, or fat. Each of these food types is a *macronutrient*. Macronutrients are the muscle in your diet. They supply your energy and support the health and generation of your tissues.

As you eat and burn off the macronutrients you consume throughout the day, your body releases two hormones, cortisol and insulin. The amount and balance of these hormones play a huge role in determining the health of you and your immune system.

> **DEFINITION**
>
> **Macronutrients** are the carbohydrates, proteins, and fats that are the core of what you eat and that support energy and tissues.

Considering Cortisol

When you haven't eaten for a while, your body becomes starved for energy. Your body enters starvation mode readily, so most likely, you're not experiencing actual starvation when this happens. However, your body does engage in an important activity during this time: it releases cortisol to break down your tissues into energy, rather than burning fuel from food. These tissues include stored fat, muscle that stores protein, and glycogen in your liver and cells, which can be released as carbohydrates. Ultimately, any of these can be converted into blood sugar for the body to use as energy.

Cortisol is often called the main stress hormone of the body. In addition to breaking down tissues for energy stores, cortisol is an immune suppressant, so having an excess of it in your system is not the best thing. Cortisol also is known to increase the percentage of fat stored in the belly, worsen your cholesterol, be toxic to neurons and cells in the brain, and because it raises blood sugar, even increase your risk of diabetes.

Managing Your Insulin

Insulin, on the other hand, is released when you eat and have an excess of energy. The body absorbs food into your tissues, storing the excess energy as fat, muscle, and carbohydrates for later use. Having too much insulin will increase fat deposition. This increases obesity, which can weaken your immune system. Having excess fat on the body, in addition to contributing to inactivity, is actually pro-inflammatory, so the body's usual immune defenses are distracted while they deal with the excess fat. Therefore, having too much insulin is also not good for your health or your immune system.

Estimating Your Caloric Needs

You want to eat an appropriate amount of food to fulfill the body's needs and not be in excess or starvation. Estimating your body's needs can be difficult, though, because people all have a different metabolism. Your needs will also vary by age, weight, activity level, and percentage of muscle. There are many online calculators that estimate your body's energy needs, measured in calories. One such free tool is available from the Mayo Clinic at mayoclinic.com/health/calorie-calculator/NU00598 (see the following figure).

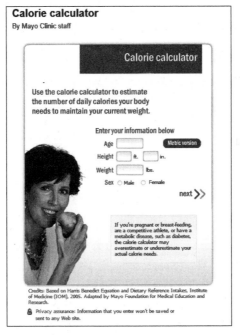

The Mayo Clinic calorie calculator.

Once you know the number of calories your body needs, you can calculate your calories by looking at food labels and seeing the estimate of calories for everything you eat, or you can calculate them based on the number of calories that are in carbohydrates, protein, and fat. Carbohydrates and protein each have 4 calories per gram, while fat has more than twice the energy with 9 calories per gram—one of the reasons excess fat intake can more easily lead to caloric excess and weight gain.

Ultimately, the key to boosting your immunity through the food you eat is to eat wholesome foods in a way that also balances your cortisol and insulin levels. Carbohydrates, protein, and fat all influence these hormone levels, as you'll read later in this chapter. By understanding how each of these affects your hormones and immune system, you can in eat in a way to support your immune strength.

Carbohydrates and the Immune System

Carbohydrates play an important role in cortisol and insulin production because it's mainly blood sugar that determines how the body releases these two vital hormones. To balance these two hormones, you not only want to make sure to eat an appropriate amount of carbohydrates at the right intervals, but you also want to try to avoid eating foods that will cause a quick spike in blood sugar levels and therefore more rapid fluctuations of your cortisol and insulin levels.

Though there are many different theories on the ideal amount of carbohydrates, it is generally recommended that they should make up about half of your daily servings of food. Before you load up that plate of pasta, however, you need to know a little more about the type of carbohydrates you eat, as not all carbohydrates are created equal. The following sections describe the two types of carbohydrates—simple and complex—and offer advice on how to measure the value of your intake.

Avoiding Simple Carbohydrates

Simple carbohydrates are foods that contain one or two nonlinked sugar compounds, such as starchy vegetables, certain fruits, sweets, processed grains, and pasta. Simple carbohydrates often taste sweeter. Because of their simple makeup and not having linked bonds that need to be broken down by the body, these carbohydrates are absorbed quickly and rapidly raise your blood sugar, giving you a so-called "sugar high."

When you eat simple carbohydrates, the abrupt rise in blood sugar levels causes your insulin levels to increase sharply to lower your blood sugar levels. So just as suddenly as the sugar high takes hold, the sugar crash—the effect when elevated insulin levels cause your blood sugar to plummet—follows. When your blood sugar levels become very low and your body needs to increase its fuel supply of sugar, your cortisol production kicks in. These yo-yo effects are harmful to your immune system because of how these hormones impair immune functioning. But they are also very harmful for your general health.

IMMUNITY ALERT

Elevated sugar, cortisol, and insulin levels are all risk factors for diabetes and cardiovascular disease, which can lead to a heart attack or stroke. For this reason, simple carbohydrates should be a very small amount of your food intake.

Eating Complex Carbohydrates

Complex carbohydrates are a much better food choice than simple carbohydrates. They contain more links than simple carbohydrates, which means that the body takes more time to break them up. As a result, cortisol and insulin swings are not as sharp, which is much better for your overall and immune health.

Complex carbohydrates include whole grains, fruits, and vegetables with high fiber content, such as apples, broccoli, and leafy green vegetables. Most fiber is not absorbed by the body; therefore, it doesn't increase your blood sugar levels at all or affect these hormones. In addition, fiber stimulates colonic health, which helps support the immune system.

Since fiber doesn't get absorbed, the body still needs carbohydrate fuel. But if some of your carbohydrates are in the form of fiber, you absorb fewer carbohydrates at once, causing less of a swing in your insulin and cortisol levels.

The following lists some high-fiber carbohydrates you should have in your diet.

High-fiber fruits:

- Apples
- Avocados
- Bananas
- Berries
- Dried fruits (such as apricots, figs, prunes, and raisins)
- Kiwi
- Oranges
- Pears

High-fiber vegetables:

- Avocados
- Beans
- Broccoli
- Brussels sprouts
- Cabbage
- Carrots
- Chickpeas (garbanzo beans)
- Eggplant
- Greens (such as collards, kale, mustard greens, Swiss chard, and turnip greens)
- Lima beans

- Mushrooms
- Peas
- Peppers
- Spinach
- Sweet potatoes
- Yams

Other high-fiber foods:

- Bran
- Legumes (beans and peanuts)
- Nuts
- Whole-grain bread
- Whole-grain pasta

Simple or Complex? Using the Glycemic Index

Many foods have a combination of simple and complex carbohy-drates. To determine how rapidly a certain food will raise your blood sugar levels, you simply need to look up its glycemic index (GI) score. You can easily find the GI scores for the 100 most common foods at health.harvard.edu/newsweek/Glycemic_index_and_ glycemic_load_for_100_foods.htm. The GI of a carbohydrate is a measure of its simplicity, or how quickly it causes a rise in insulin or sugar.

The following are some basic guidelines:

- A low GI score is 55 and under.
- A medium GI score is 56 to 69.
- A high GI score is 70 and above.

In general, simple carbohydrates, which you should avoid as much as possible, have a high GI. Complex carbohydrates, which increase insulin and sugar levels more slowly, have a low GI.

The following are some foods with a high GI score:

- Baked goods
- Low-fiber cereals
- Pasta
- Rice
- White bread

Foods with a low GI score include the following:

- Fruits
- Legumes
- Nonstarchy vegetables
- Whole and minimally processed grains

IMMUNITY ALERT

How you prepare your food greatly affects its nutritional value. If you fry food that has a low GI score, you negate any benefit the raw food offers.

Protein and the Immune System

Proteins are a part of all the cells in your body. They consist of 20 types of amino acids, including essential amino acids, which you must get from food in order for your cells to thrive. Amino acids are commonly called the "building blocks" of protein.

The protein in your cells is constantly cycled as your body burns energy. When you consume protein in food, that protein replenishes the protein that has been used up, enabling your cells to flourish. As you can imagine, protein is an important part of a healthy diet. Your protein needs may vary, depending on your activity levels, as protein is the key component to muscles that are constantly rebuilding in active people.

Now, just to complicate things a little further, some protein sources are *complete proteins*—they contain all 20 amino acids. These include mostly protein from animal sources, such as meat and dairy. Others are *complementary proteins*, meaning they are short of one or two amino acids and need to be combined with another protein source to make a complete protein. These include mostly protein from nonanimal sources, such as vegetables and grains.

IMMUNE BOOSTER

Two proteins from nonanimal sources can be combined to create one complete protein. For example, beans and rice form a complete protein.

Because of protein's importance, it should comprise 10 to 35 percent of your daily caloric intake. The trick is to be sure you're consuming the best protein. Many protein sources are laden with bad fats, such as saturated and trans fats. A common source of protein is animal meat, but many meats are laden with saturated fat that's bad for your immune system and overall health (we discuss fat more in the next section). Healthy proteins, on the other hand, have little fat or mainly healthy unsaturated fats.

Good sources of protein include the following:

- Eggs
- Some fruits, including avocados, berries, and dried fruits
- Lean chicken or beef
- Legumes, such as beans and peanuts
- Low-fat milk and other low-fat dairy products
- Nuts and seeds, such as pumpkin and sunflower seeds
- Processed soy protein, such as tofu
- Salmon, tuna, and other fish that have good types of fats
- Vegetables such as artichokes, asparagus, broccoli, Brussels sprouts, cauliflower, and watercress
- Whole, unrefined grains such as barley, bran, bulgur, whole oats, quinoa, and whole-wheat pasta

Fat and the Immune System

Fats carry more than twice as many calories per gram as carbohydrates. Fat is a secondary use of energy in the body after carbohydrates, so in addition to containing more calories, fats are much more prone to being stored in the body as excess weight. Excess fat is proinflammatory, which weakens your immune system. So what's the upside to fats?

Well, certain types of fats are essential for cellular and tissue development. These include unsaturated fats, especially omega-3 fatty acids, which are commonly found in fish. These fats have been shown to increase immune health and also support good cardiovascular health. Eggs, flaxseed, and avocados are excellent sources of omega-3 fatty acids.

IMMUNE BOOSTER

If you have an aversion to fish and need to boost your omega-3s, try taking fish oil or flax oil supplements, as described in Chapter 12.

As for how much fat is too much fat, some fats are saturated fats or trans fats and are not considered an essential part of a nutritional diet. They are considered "extras" and should be avoided when possible.

Fats to avoid include the following:

- Beef fat
- Butter
- Chicken fat
- Milk fat
- Partially hydrogenated oil
- Pork fat (lard)
- Shortening
- Stick margarine

A good but not perfect rule of thumb to remember where good and bad fats come from is to think in terms of the food source. If the food source is plant based, a fish, or an egg, you're looking at a good fat. If the food source is animal based (chicken, beef, or pork), the fat is saturated. Look for lean cuts of these meats—you'll get your protein without an excess of bad fat. Oils that are solid at room temperature, such as margarine and shortening, are high in trans fats and should be avoided.

> **IMMUNE BOOSTER**
>
> What your meat eats matters. According to the Department of Food Science in Melbourne, Australia, grass-fed beef has a higher omega-3 fatty acid content than regular beef, which has virtually none.

For optimal nutritional health, limit your overall fat intake to 20 grams per day, and minimize the amount of saturated fat that makes up those 20 grams. Remember, good overall health means good immune health.

The Effects of Other Additives on Your Immune System

Although carbohydrates, protein, and fat tend to be the largest component of what you eat and have the most direct influence on your immune system, plenty of other components of food that you ingest affect your immunity as well. Most people consume other additives to food and beverages, including preservatives, artificial sweeteners, and caffeine. All of these can affect your immune system in various ways, so it's essential to understand and manage how you eat to boost your immunity.

Preservatives

Artificial substances are used in just about all processed foods. Not all artificial substances have been directly studied, but we do know that substances the body did not evolve to process causes inflammation. Chronic inflammation, of course, hurts your immune system and long-term health.

Because so many chemicals are used in food processing, it's impossible to know them all. But the following are some of the most commonly used preservatives:

- Sulfur dioxide, a bleach used to conceal or prevent brown spots in produce
- Sodium benzoate (also called *benzoic acid*), which is found in soft drinks, fruit juice, and margarine
- Nitrates and nitrites, which are used for bacon, hot dogs, and lunch meats
- Sulfites, sulfur dioxide, and metabisulfites, which stop fungus from growing

Some people have allergic reactions to these chemicals, which can be severe. In general, you want to avoid consuming preservatives. This also applies to things that are "natural" but consumed in far more excessive amounts than we evolved to consume, such as caffeine (discussed later in this chapter).

Artificial Sweeteners

Although using artificial sweeteners can help limit your intake of calories and make managing diabetes a little easier, using these additives is a source of great controversy. It doesn't help that many of the studies on adverse effects of the chemicals on the body conflict with one another. For example, some studies show that artificial sweeteners are linked to cancer, but just as many (if not more) show that they are not. You can find many claims that these additives actually cause weight gain, but frankly, the science just isn't in on that just yet.

The following are the most commonly used artificial sweeteners:

- Aspartame (Equal, NutraSweet)
- Saccharin (SugarTwin, Sweet'N Low)
- Sucralose (Splenda)

The most common, and most controversial, artificial sweetener is aspartame. The following are some foods that contain aspartame and the amount they contain:

- 12-oz. diet soft drinks: up to 225 mg of aspartame
- 8-oz. yogurt: 80 mg of aspartame
- 1 packet of Equal: 22 mg of aspartame

The FDA has set the acceptable daily intake (ADI) for aspartame at 50 mg/kg (milligrams per kilogram) of body weight. Of course this involves math, right? It's not so bad. To determine your ADI, all you have to do is divide your weight in pounds by 2.2 and then multiply the result by 50. So if you weigh 160 pounds, your weight in kilograms would be 73 (160 ÷ 2.2), and your ADI for aspartame would be 3,650 mg (50 × 73). As you can see, that's quite a few diet soft drinks.

The ADI for saccharin is 5 mg/kg of body weight. To determine your ADI, follow the same process as for the aspartame calculation. Divide your weight in pounds by 2.2 and then multiply it by 5. For example, if you weighed 160 pounds, your weight in kilograms would be 73 (160 ÷ 2.2), and your ADI for saccharin would be 365 mg (5 × 73).

IMMUNITY ALERT

For many years, saccharin was thought to cause cancer. This has since been disproven, and the FDA has officially removed the warning information from the product.

Sucralose was the subject of much scrutiny, but based on animal and human studies, the FDA has deemed it safe for human consumption. The ADI for sucralose is 5 mg/kg of body weight/day. To determine your ADI, simply divide your weight in pounds by 2.2 and then multiply it by 50. For example, if you weigh 200 pounds, your weight in kilograms would be 91 (200 ÷ 2.2), and your ADI for sucralose would be 455 mg (91 × 5).

If you use an artificial sweetener instead of excessive amounts of sugar, you may lose weight due to the reduced calories, which has health benefits. Therefore, on occasion, the benefit of these artificial sweeteners may outweigh the risk. Of course, the ideal is to lose the weight without using artificial sweeteners, but for some, artificial sweeteners represent a ready option for losing excess weight and reducing obesity. Therefore, the decision to use these products is a personal one based on the risk and benefit of these various options. The science is still coming in, so you really must determine the benefit you gain and, as always, practice moderation.

Caffeine and Energy Inducers

Energy inducers, such as caffeine and the other chemicals found in energy drinks, generally function by increasing the body's release of cortisol to increase blood sugar and therefore your energy levels. Remember, however, that cortisol is an immune suppressant and causes other negative health effects when chronically elevated.

In other words, caffeine and other energy inducers tend to have a harmful effect on the immune system. In terms of recommended intake, the less you consume, the better for your immune system. Giving up such substances can be hard, as your body can develop dependence to them and therefore go through withdrawal if quitting too abruptly.

To be successful in giving up caffeine and other energy supplements, decrease them in a step-wise fashion. Start consuming less with each drink or spread out the times you drink them further and further. To create more energy, exercise in the morning and move around whenever you feel your energy is starting to become low. If you drink coffee, simulate the activity by putting water in a coffee mug, which will also help you keep hydrated. If you develop a headache, over-the-counter products such as acetaminophen and ibuprofen should help.

Eventually, your body will adjust to the change and your symptoms will improve. The biggest difference though is your body will be healthier and your immune system will become stronger.

Not Just *What* You Eat, But *How*

The foods you eat are a significant factor in determining your overall and immune health. The way you structure your meals, your portion sizes, and the exact foods you eat are equally important. The following are some basic guidelines to help you make good decisions when structuring your meals.

First, eat the optimal amounts your body needs, not too much or too little.

> **IMMUNE BOOSTER**
>
> If you need help determining the optimal amounts of food your body needs, visit choosemyplate.gov, which is a great resource for all things nutrition.

Make sure you also balance your cortisol and insulin levels. Eat frequent small meals as opposed to spaced-out large meals, which cause larger cortisol and insulin swings.

Also, eat slightly more in the evening than you do early in the day, as the longest time your body goes without food is during the night when you are sleeping, and your body enters starvation mode. Cortisol levels are highest in the morning until you consume breakfast and "break" the "fast."

Finally, get back to basics. People's bodies evolved with certain diets over tens of thousands of years, and it appears that diets consistent with the foods of our ancestors are healthful. Eat lean (unfried) meats, fish, nuts, produce, and whole grains.

Our ancestors were constantly faced with sources of infection and stressors on their bodies, so having a good immune system was important. By eating the way our ancestors ate—whole, unprocessed foods—you can boost your immunity the same way they did. We evolved to survive on these foods, so our bodies are naturally programmed to respond well to them. This sort of diet promotes our long-term health, energy, and mood, all of which benefits the immune system.

Over the last two decades, "paleo" diets have become increasingly popular because it embraces the philosophy of eating based on what we have evolved to eat to promote good health, and believe eating in such a fashion can support our immunity. By understanding how what we eat affects our immune system, you can consider whether eating "paleo" or other variants is right for you.

The Least You Need to Know

- Aim for lean protein, complex carbohydrates, and unsaturated fats for immune and total body health.
- Minimize artificial substances and energy inducers that promote inflammation and immune suppression.
- Smaller balanced meals will lead to more stable hormone levels and provide greater support to your immune system.

Vitamins and Minerals: More than Essential

In This Chapter

- Vitamin D: the sunshine vitamin
- Antioxidants and the fruits and vegetables loaded with them
- Does vitamin C truly boost immunity?
- Zinc and its ability to shorten the duration of the common cold
- Other vitamins and minerals that can potentially boost your immunity

For centuries, society has searched for ways to prevent or cure illnesses. Many vitamins and minerals have been thought to do just that.

But of the many studied, only a few have been shown to be effective for immunity. Though the fact that so many don't work may be disheartening, it is very exciting that several do. In this chapter, we look at vitamins and minerals and their potential benefits to your immunity.

Vitamin D

No supplement has received more attention in recent years than vitamin D. Through genetic expression, it has been associated with immunity, inflammation, cardiovascular disease, and much more.

Many people tend to be deficient in vitamin D. You can therefore potentially improve your immunity and lower your risk of many diseases by increasing your vitamin D levels.

The Many Effects of Vitamin D

Vitamin D has been shown in numerous studies to affect many of the body's processes, including genetic expression. For example, vitamin D controls the expression of various genes that influence your physiology, which significantly impacts your immunity and risk of long-term or chronic diseases. Vitamin D also controls the genetic expression of various immune factors. As you read earlier in this book, in addition to fighting infections, a strong immune system can help suppress abnormal tumor cells, and vitamin D has actually been shown to directly influence the expression of tumor cells. Therefore, optimal vitamin D levels can potentially reduce your risk of cancer.

Vitamin D levels have also been closely associated with inflammation. Studies have shown that vitamin D levels closely correlate with inflammation. As you'll recall from previous chapters, inflammation is associated with cardiovascular disease, cancer, dementia, and many other chronic diseases. So by lowering your inflammation, you can reduce your future risk of these devastating diseases.

IMMUNE BOOSTER

In research studies, it has been shown that increasing vitamin D levels lowers certain markers of inflammation, most notably C-reactive protein (CRP).

However, like all dietary adjustments and supplementation, this beneficial effect was only seen up to a point. Studies found inflammation actually increased when vitamin D levels were extremely high. This suggests that vitamin D has an optimal level at which it's effective, though this level can vary by person. Later in this chapter, we discuss how to know your optimal level.

Primary Sources of Vitamin D

Vitamin D is known as the "sunshine vitamin" because the sun is the primary source of vitamin D for most people. In fact, it is estimated that for many people who receive only casual sun exposure (meaning they don't make an active effort to get sun exposure), almost 90 percent of their vitamin D is received from the sun.

> **IMMUNITY ALERT**
>
> To be precise, the sun doesn't actually give you vitamin D—rather, sunlight causes a chemical reaction in your skin, which results in the production of vitamin D in your body.

Vitamin D has other sources, though. Some foods contain vitamin D naturally or are fortified with it. Natural foods that contain vitamin D include animals that have high levels of vitamin D themselves, such as fish. And, although the beneficial effects of vitamin D have only been recently discovered, dairy foods have been fortified with vitamin D for many years because vitamin D has long been known to facilitate the absorption of calcium, which is common in dairy-based products.

You can also get vitamin D through supplementation. Because of its calcium-absorption properties, for years vitamin D was commonly taken by older people who wanted to increase their bone strength to treat or prevent osteoporosis. However, more recent knowledge concerning vitamin D deficiency has expanded its use beyond that. Vitamin D can be found as part of a multivitamin—for example, a combined vitamin D and calcium supplement—or as a standalone supplement.

Why People Are Deficient in Vitamin D

As mentioned earlier in this section, the primary source of vitamin D is the sun. Our ancestors spent most of their waking hours outdoors, with lots of exposure to the sun. Unfortunately, most people today don't get nearly as much sunlight, so their vitamin D levels tend to be lower than they are evolved to have. In fact, it is estimated that more than 50 percent of people are deficient in vitamin D.

This deficiency in vitamin D can have harmful effects on your immune health, as well as potentially increase your risk of cancer and heart disease. I use the word *potentially* because these diseases often take many decades to develop. Also, our knowledge of vitamin D's genetic effects is relatively recent, so a direct relation between adjusting vitamin D levels and future incidence of disease can't actually be verified. Instead we use blood tests, such as inflammatory biomarkers like hs-CRP, to try and identify whether adjusting our vitamin D level may affect our future risk of disease.

No one knows the optimal amount of sun exposure for vitamin D. Clearly, more is not always better because of risks of overexposure, most notably skin cancer. Also, even though many people have a vitamin D deficiency, the amount of sunlight necessary to increase vitamin D levels differs by individual. Research recommendations vary, but many suggest somewhere between 10 and 30 minutes of peak-time sun exposure (10 A.M. to 3 P.M.) a day to attain the maximum amount of sunlight while minimizing the risk of UV damage from prolonged exposure. And, fortunately, there are ways to identify the best levels of vitamin D for you personally.

Knowing and Improving Your Vitamin D

The decision to increase vitamin D levels, as well as what level to increase them to, is an individual one. Though some increase in vitamin D will likely benefit most people, to determine exactly how much requires added information. As mentioned previously, researchers have shown that extremely high levels of vitamin D can actually increase inflammation, so it's possible to get too much vitamin D (see Chapter 4 for more information about the effects of inflammation on your immune system).

Your physician can test your levels of vitamin D—or more specially, 25-OH vitamin D, the precursor to the vitamin D that the body uses—to identify if your vitamin D levels are low. Your doctor can also check your levels of inflammation, such as CRP, via a separate test (see Chapter 4 for more on CRP). The two can then be repeated and correlated to identify the vitamin D level that produces the lowest CRP. Not all physicians perform such testing regularly, so if your doctor is unable or unwilling to perform such testing, you can seek out physicians who perform such wellness testing through a service, such as WellnessFX (wellnessfx.com). Testing helps you not only identify your level of vitamin D deficiency, but also gives you an idea of how much you can increase your vitamin D intake based on your inflammation levels.

If testing identifies a vitamin D deficiency, you can boost your levels in several ways. One way is to increase your sun exposure incrementally. If you decide to do this, studies recommend that you spend short periods of time (10 to 30 minutes) outside more frequently rather than spend long periods of time outside less frequently to minimize the risk of sunburn and skin cancer.

Another option is to increase your intake of vitamin D–fortified foods. As mentioned previously, the richest sources of vitamin D tend to be fish and dairy products. Both are also great sources of other beneficial immune boosters beyond vitamin D—for fish, it's omega-3 fatty acids; for dairy products, it's calcium. Of course, you can only consume so much fish and milk, and some people with certain diet restrictions may not be able to consume any at all. The final option, after increasing sun exposure and vitamin D in your diet, is supplementation.

Many supplements exist as a standalone product or as part of other vitamins and supplements. The National Institute of Health Office of Dietary Supplements recommends adults consume at least 600 IUs (International Units), or 15 mg, of vitamin D daily.

Antioxidants

Antioxidants represent a group of vitamins and minerals that act in similar ways to protect the body from free radicals. The main antioxidants include vitamins A, C, and E; zinc; and selenium. You will learn more about these later in the chapter; for now, we'll look at antioxidants in general.

DEFINITION

Antioxidants are elements that bind free radicals—which are thought to contribute to the aging process—that are produced through oxidation reactions in the body.

What Do Antioxidants Do?

Antioxidants earned their name because they attempt to reverse oxidation in the body. Many of the body's usual physiological reactions result in unstable particles known as *free radicals*. When our body cells use oxygen, they naturally produce free radicals (by-products), which can cause damage. It is believed free radicals play a significant role in the overall aging process and contribute to many chronic diseases, including atherosclerosis in cardiovascular disease and mutations in cancer. Free radicals have also been implicated in hindering the immune system.

Antioxidants help bind and eliminate these free radicals, in theory preventing them from doing some of their damage. The best sources of antioxidants are fruits and vegetables, and it is well established that people with diets high in fruits and vegetables have a lower prevalence of many chronic diseases. Many scientists believe this is due to the antioxidants in them and therefore recommend eating more fruits and vegetables to improve immune function.

The ideal way to get antioxidants is through natural food, as the nutrients seem to be most effective in their natural state (see Chapter 11 for more on antioxidant-rich foods).

Sources of Antioxidants and Supplementation

The best sources of antioxidants are plants, especially fruits and vegetables. Certain foods are rich sources of multiple antioxidants. For example, many dark, leafy greens are rich sources of vitamins A and E, while many tropical fruit are rich sources of vitamins C and E. (These immune-boosting foods are discussed more in Chapter 11, and recipes using them are provided in Chapters 13 and 14.)

As with other nutrients, when you're unable to obtain enough antioxidants through food, you can take supplements. Though taking supplements of individual antioxidants can be helpful, you might consider taking a combination supplement, such as a general multivitamin or a combination of antioxidants. Taking a combination supplement helps you avoid having a deficiency in a single vitamin while not providing so much of one that it leads to toxicity.

Vitamin C

Vitamin C is the most traditional supplement to boost immunity. For years, people have taken vitamin C to prevent infection and to try to decrease the duration and severity of illness. Its origins as an immune booster are due to citric juices, such as orange juice, being used by people as a home remedy. And because of its long-standing popularity, much research exists into whether the plethora of vitamin C supplements actually support immunity.

Are the Immune Effects True?

Studies have been performed to analyze whether vitamin C has immune-boosting effects prior to or during infection. Sadly, vitamin C has not been shown to be clearly effective in improving immunity, so most scientists have come to the conclusion that vitamin C is not necessarily an immune booster.

Vitamin C is an antioxidant, though, and as discussed previously, antioxidants may have certain value in our health. In addition, while vitamin C has not been shown to necessarily strengthen the immune system, many people say they feel better when they take vitamin C during an infection, and there may be a logical reason for this.

Vitamin C is a weak acid that's otherwise known as *ascorbic acid*. Though acids in general aren't healthy to consume, ascorbic acid is weak enough that it doesn't have significantly harmful effects on the body unless taken in doses hundreds of times the U.S. Recommended Daily Allowance (RDA). Despite being a weak acid, it can potentially have acid activity on what it contacts directly. For example, some people may have stomach discomfort when consuming vitamin C because of how the acid interacts directly with the stomach. Similarly, vitamin C can help soothe a sore throat because the acid interacts directly with the bacteria in the throat. It's for this reason that citric juices like orange juice feel soothing on the throat and are a traditional home remedy.

IMMUNITY ALERT

You can minimize stomach discomfort from ingesting vitamin C by taking sodium ascorbate or calcium ascorbate.

Therefore, it's okay to take vitamin C if it helps you feel better when you are sick. However, vitamin C likely doesn't have any major effect on the immune system.

Sources of Vitamin C and Supplementation

The best sources of vitamin C are citric fruits and juices, with the most popular being orange juice. If you're getting sick of drinking glass after glass of orange juice, though, you can get your vitamin C from many other fruits and vegetables. Some of these sources include the following:

- Brussels sprouts
- Cantaloupe
- Grapefruit
- Green pepper
- Guava
- Kiwi
- Red pepper
- Strawberries

In addition to vitamin C, these fruits and vegetables are packed with other vitamins and offer your system valuable hydration. Therefore, even if they're not directly immune boosting, they can be soothing and great for your health.

While it's tough to consume multiple servings of many of these options, fortunately, you can make them into juice. Even if juicing, though, sometimes it can be difficult to consume multiple servings of vitamin C–rich foods. In this case, an acceptable alternative is supplementation.

Because of vitamin C's longtime popularity and folklore as an immune booster, many different types of vitamin C supplements exist, ranging from pills, to lozenges, to even dissolvable fizzy powder. All are equally acceptable supplements, and the quicker the vitamin dissolves, the quicker it will be absorbed by your system. However, it's unclear whether faster absorption leads to greater effectiveness.

Recommendations for doses of vitamin C vary, but the following table provides some general recommendations from the National Institute of Health Office of Dietary Supplements.

Recommended Daily Allowances (RDAs) for Vitamin C

Age	Male	Female	Pregnancy	Lactation
0 to 6 months	40 mg	40 mg		
7 to 12 months	50 mg	50 mg		
1 to 3 years	15 mg	15 mg		
4 to 8 years	25 mg	25 mg		
9 to 13 years	45 mg	45 mg		
14 to 18 years	75 mg	65 mg	80 mg	115 mg
19+ years	90 mg	75 mg	85 mg	120 mg

Extremely high doses of vitamin C have not been shown to be harmful beyond some mild gastrointestinal effects, such as upset stomach and diarrhea. Regardless, all vitamin C supplement warnings should be reviewed and, if you have any concerns, discussed with your physician.

> **IMMUNITY ALERT**
>
> Always consider food for nutrition before trying a supplement. Supplementation is for when it's not possible to get the desired amount of a nutrient through just food.

Vitamins A and E

Vitamins A and E are the two most popular antioxidants. Though both are antioxidants, like all antioxidants, they have many key benefits that are different from one another.

How Vitamins A and E Can Help Your Immunity

Vitamin A is essential for vision. A deficiency in vitamin A can lead to a condition known as night blindness, where it's difficult or impossible to see in low light. Vitamin A comes in the diet primarily in two forms: retinol and carotene. Retinol is more commonly found in animal products such as meats, fish, milk, and cheese, while carotene is more commonly in fruits and vegetables. There are different types of carotene as well, with the most popular known as beta-carotene. All of these forms of vitamin A in the diet are converted to vitamin A in the body.

In addition to its activity in vision, because of its antioxidant activity, vitamin A is recommended to aid immune function and decrease your risk of future chronic diseases. Furthermore, vitamin A has been shown to be a key ingredient in the development of cells, including immune cells.

The following are the intake recommendations for vitamin A by the National Institute of Health Office of Dietary Supplements:

Recommended Daily Allowances (RDAs) for Vitamin A

Age	Male	Female	Pregnancy	Lactation
0 to 6 months	400 mcg RAE	400 mcg RAE		
7 to 12 months	500 mcg RAE	500 mcg RAE		
1 to 3 years	300 mcg RAE	300 mcg RAE		
4 to 8 years	400 mcg RAE	400 mcg RAE		
9 to 13 years	600 mcg RAE	600 mcg RAE		
14 to 18 years	900 mcg RAE	700 mcg RAE	750 mcg RAE	1,200 mcg RAE
19 to 50 years	900 mcg RAE	700 mcg RAE	770 mcg RAE	1,300 mcg RAE
51+ years	900 mcg RAE	700 mcg RAE		

Notice the recommendations increase with age—especially for men—and due to pregnancy or lactation. However, know that too much vitamin A may be a bad thing. Excess vitamin A has been associated with neurological symptoms, including blurred vision, dizziness, headache, and even excess fluid and pressure around the brain. These symptoms typically require consumption of at least 10 times the recommended dose of vitamin A, and often more, to occur.

IMMUNE BOOSTER

For people over 70 years old, the recommended dosage of vitamin A is increased to 800 IUs, or 20 mg, due to the need for increased absorption of calcium to help prevent or treat osteoporosis.

Vitamin E comes in various forms known as tocopherols and tocotrienols. Vitamin E has been shown in laboratory studies of cells to have immune-modulating effects. In addition, like other antioxidants, vitamin E is believed to reduce signs of aging, ranging from chronic diseases to skin deterioration. In certain studies, vitamin E has even been shown to reduce bad cholesterol, leading to less cardiovascular disease. Vitamin E has also been shown to reduce the risk of certain cancers and even possibly slow the rate of cognitive decline in dementia. These effects are believed to be due to its antioxidant activity.

Vitamin E deficiency is quite rare, as many foods contain vitamin E. But when a deficiency does exist, it has been shown to increase the risk of infections. Vitamin E toxicity is also not typically seen.

IMMUNE BOOSTER

A diverse diet of fruits, vegetables, meat, and dairy can help ensure a balanced intake of antioxidants as well as decrease the risk of vitamin deficiency.

Sources of Vitamins A and E and Supplementation

The very best sources of vitamin A include the following:

- Apricots
- Beef liver
- Butternut squash
- Cantaloupe
- Carrots
- Cayenne pepper
- Chili pepper
- Dark, leafy greens
- Paprika
- Sweet potatoes

The best sources of vitamin E include the following:

- Broccoli
- Collard greens
- Kale

- Nuts
- Red bell pepper
- Spinach
- Tropical fruit, such as apricots, mango, and papaya
- Vegetable oils, such as olive oil
- Wheat

If you can't obtain enough of these vitamins through food, you can always take supplements. Try to take a combination supplement to make sure you get enough of them and still avoid potentially toxic levels.

Zinc

Zinc has recently become the most popular supplement to take during an illness. For hundreds of years, people have been searching for medications to cure the common cold, and while nothing has been found to do so, zinc has come close. Numerous studies have shown that zinc can decrease the duration and severity of the common cold.

Zinc and the Immune System

Zinc serves many functions in the body; it has been identified as a key part of over 100 physiologic reactions. These reactions range from cellular production, to wound healing, to immune function.

For some time, zinc deficiency has been associated with immune deficiency, believed to be due to poor production of immune cells. More recently, interest has been focused on whether higher amounts of zinc could enhance immunity. Zinc has been long known to be an antioxidant, but the proposed strengthening of immunity that zinc could provide goes beyond its antioxidant activity.

IMMUNE BOOSTER

Despite decades of research, zinc is the first supplement to have consistent evidence showing it decreases the duration and severity of the common cold.

Many studies have been performed to assess the effect of zinc on the common cold. As with any research, there have been multiple findings, but the analysis of all the research in aggregate suggests that if taken at the right time and in the right way, zinc does reduce the duration and severity of the common cold. In addition, some research suggests that increased zinc intake chronically can lead to reduced incidence of colds.

It's believed that zinc reduces the virulence of the common cold by attaching to certain cellular receptors that block the binding of the cold virus to the cell, decreasing the virus's ability to replicate. Also, it is thought that most of this interference of replication occurs in the nasal mucosa, where cold viruses replicate the most.

Because of this mechanism, only zinc taken early in an illness has the opportunity to bind cellular receptors before the cold virus does. If zinc is started after the first 24 hours, though, typically the cold virus has had a chance to replicate almost fully.

Sources of Zinc and Supplementation

Like all nutrients, zinc can be obtained through food. Few foods contain very high amounts of zinc, with certain exceptions. The following table includes a few of the highest-concentration zinc foods with their respective milligrams per serving, according to information from the National Institute of Health Office of Dietary Supplements.

Selected Food Sources of Zinc

Food	Milligrams (mg) per Serving
Oysters, cooked, breaded, and fried, 3 ounces	74.0
Beef chuck roast, braised, 3 ounces	7.0
Alaskan king crab, cooked, 3 ounces	6.5
Beef patty, broiled, 3 ounces	5.3
Breakfast cereal, fortified with 25 percent of the DV for zinc, ¾-cup serving	3.8

Because many foods do not contain high amounts of zinc, supplementation with zinc is very common.

The very first popular "cold" supplement to contain zinc was a brand called Cold-Eeze. Cold-Eeze quickly became very popular because many users began to swear by how the zinc-containing throat lozenges reduced the length and severity of their colds.

Many other forms of zinc supplements are now on the market as well—including zinc tablets, nasal swabs, and gels—but the best studied are still zinc lozenges. The type of zinc shown to be the most effective with the least amount of side effects is zinc gluconate. When picking a zinc supplement, look for zinc gluconate among the ingredients.

IMMUNITY ALERT

Because of the belief that zinc might interfere with nasal replication, several topical nasal zinc supplements have been put on the market. These seem to have similar effectiveness to lozenges, but there have been case reports of these topical applications causing a loss of the ability to smell, or anosmia. Therefore, taking zinc lozenges may be better due to their lower risks.

The following is the recommended intake of zinc for various ages from the National Institute of Health Office of Dietary Supplements:

Recommended Daily Allowances (RDAs) for Zinc

Age	Male	Female	Pregnancy	Lactation
0 to 6 months	2 mg	2 mg		
7 to 12 months	3 mg	3 mg		
1 to 3 years	3 mg	3 mg		
4 to 8 years	5 mg	5 mg		
9 to 13 years	8 mg	8 mg		
14 to 18 years	11 mg	9 mg	12 mg	13 mg
19+ years	11 mg	8 mg	11 mg	12 mg

As is common with many supplements, need for zinc increases with age and due to pregnancy and lactation. However, female needs actually decrease slightly once they are past puberty.

For zinc to be effective, supplementation should begin within the first 24 hours after the onset of an illness to be able to interfere with viral replication. Recommended doses during active illness are at least 13 mg of zinc every few hours.

Certain substances, when ingested within 30 minutes before or after a zinc supplement, may interfere with the absorption of zinc. These substances include fiber, soy protein, iron, and citric juices. In addition, zinc can interact and interfere with many medications. The most notable of these medications is antibiotics, which many who are ill are taking. Therefore, it's important before taking a zinc supplement to research and ask your physician about the potential interaction of zinc with other medications.

More Vitamins and Minerals

The vitamins and minerals discussed previously comprise many of the most common that are thought to benefit immune and overall health. But other vitamins and minerals have gotten increasing scrutiny over the last few years for the benefits they might provide to your immune system.

Iron

Iron is the key component of red blood cells, which obtain oxygen from the lungs and carry it throughout the body to tissues that use oxygen for proper functioning. Without iron, none of your tissues would be viable, as they would not be able to receive essential oxygen. Because of this, iron deficiency causes many problems, including poor immunity.

Oxygen is essential to your immunity. Many of your immune factors use a reaction involving oxygen to attack infections. Also, oxygen makes your tissues stronger and more able to fight infections. Basically, oxygen is great at fighting infections. That's why when a person gets an abscess (an infection of the skin), doctors will open and pack the infection to keep it exposed to air—the oxygen suppresses any return of the infection.

Without enough iron, your body cannot circulate adequate oxygen, making you and your various tissues much more susceptible for infection. Unfortunately, many people are iron deficient. Women are at increased risk for iron deficiency due to losing iron-containing blood during menstrual periods. Athletes also have a greater chance of not having the iron supplies they need due to their increased need for oxygen at times of high activity. Certain diets low in iron-containing foods like meats or spinach may also result in not enough iron intake.

Any iron deficiency leads to anemia, or low blood count, meaning fewer blood cells are available to carry oxygen, leading to greater susceptibility to infection.

The connection between iron deficiency and anemia is not just theoretical; numerous studies have confirmed an increased susceptibility to infection in those with anemia. Therefore, in people with anemia due to iron deficiency, iron supplementation is beneficial. If you are unsure whether you are iron deficient, don't take high-dose iron supplements—too much iron intake can lead to many health problems. Either take a low-dose iron supplement, such as a multivitamin with iron, or get tested. To know if you have iron-deficiency anemia, ask your doctor to order simple blood tests.

Selenium and Copper

As with iron deficiency, selenium and copper deficiency have been shown in studies to impair the immune system. Unlike with iron, the mechanisms for how such a deficiency affects the immune system are not completely understood, though there are many theories.

Selenium and copper act as essential elements for neutrophils attacking antigens (see Chapter 1 for more on neutrophils). They also are antioxidants that protect various body systems, including your immune system, from free radicals. Regardless of how these elements influence immunity, deficiencies in selenium and copper contribute to a deficiency in the immune system.

Copper and selenium deficiency are difficult to detect. Though they can be found on blood tests, these tests are far less common and more expensive than checking for, for example, iron deficiency.

IMMUNITY ALERT

Getting tested for copper and selenium deficiency is far less common, more expensive, and difficult to access than many other vitamins and minerals because deficiency in these elements is less common.

Therefore, the safest and most effective strategy to ensure against deficiencies in copper and selenium, while not risking taking excess amounts, is to take a low dose of each as part of a comprehensive multivitamin.

B Vitamins

Many different vitamins that are considered "B vitamins" play important roles in cellular metabolism. They are each called B vitamins because they once were all thought to be one single vitamin. Together they are referred to as "B complex." Each B vitamin has its own specific name and function, and many are thought to relate to immune function. The different B vitamins and their individual functions include the following:

- B_1 (thiamine)—production of energy from carbohydrates and the synthesis of DNA and RNA, the genetic ingredients of cells
- B_2 (riboflavin)—creation of energy using various energy cycles and breaking down fatty acids for energy
- B_3 (niacin)—metabolism of sugar, alcohol, and fat
- B_5 (pantothenic acid)—oxidation of fatty acids and sugars and synthesis of protein and hormones
- B_6 (pyridoxine)—metabolism of protein and fats and production of blood sugar

- B_7 (biotin)—metabolism of fats, protein, and sugar
- B_9 (folic acid)—creation of DNA as part of cellular production through metabolism of protein and other DNA
- B_{12} (cyanocobalamin)—production of blood cells; metabolism of sugar, fat, and protein

A deficiency in any of these could theoretically have a bad effect on the immune system. But of all the B vitamins, only B_6, B_9, and B_{12} deficiency have been shown to definitively negatively affect immune function. Again, the best strategy to avoid deficiencies in B vitamins is to take a comprehensive multivitamin that contains all the essential vitamins and minerals of the immune system and overall health discussed in this chapter.

The Least You Need to Know

- Many people are vitamin D deficient, which inhibits the immune system and contributes to other chronic diseases.
- Antioxidants may benefit your immune system and reduce your risk for other chronic diseases.
- Zinc has been shown to reduce the duration and severity of the common cold.
- Consider taking a multivitamin to get a safe level of each type of vitamin that also benefits your immunity in many ways.

Immunity Superfoods

In This Chapter

- Antioxidant-rich fruits and vegetables
- The fiber boost of grains
- Protein-packed dairy, meat, and nuts
- Drinks and spices to balance your immune-boosting diet

As you learned in the previous chapter, certain nutrients can support your immunity. Though taking certain supplements is certainly reasonable if you cannot get an adequate amount of a nutrient from food, the ideal form of any nutrient is its natural form in food. By considering what foods are packed with the most nutrients, you can get the most from your diet and then supplement as necessary.

This chapter reviews some of those immunity superfoods and what nutrients those foods have that can support your immunity.

Fruits and Vegetables

Fruits and vegetables are packed with antioxidants, the nutrients that bind the free radicals generated by many of the body's reactions and implicated in many of the aging processes. These include vitamins A, C, and E and certain minerals such as zinc, selenium, and copper. Fruits and vegetables are also low in fat and offer plenty of hydration, both of which are important in general health and during infections.

Fruits and vegetables are also packed with *phytochemicals*. While certain phytochemicals and their benefits have been identified, researchers are constantly identifying new phytochemicals and their benefits. Thousands of phytochemicals have many health advantages, particularly in the reduction of your risk of cardiovascular disease, inflammation, cancer, dementia, and so on. So increasing your intake of fruits and vegetables will only benefit your health.

DEFINITION

Phytochemicals are chemical compounds that occur naturally in plants.

Broccoli and Kale

Broccoli and kale are "cruciferous," meaning they are part of the cabbage family of vegetables. All members of this family are noted for being packed with certain nutrients.

Cruciferous vegetables, especially broccoli and kale, are loaded with the antioxidants vitamins A and C. In fact, a serving of broccoli has nearly one third of an entire day's worth of the U.S. Recommended Daily Allowance (RDA) of vitamin A. Moreover, broccoli contains nearly an entire day's worth of the U.S. RDA of vitamin C. Kale has approximately 10 to 20 percent less of each nutrient but is still packed with plenty.

In addition to these antioxidants, certain other phytonutrients have been identified as immune boosters in both broccoli and kale. In fact, each has been shown to actually increase the white blood cell production of antibodies. Though the mechanisms for this immune enhancement and cancer suppression are not fully known, some of the unique nutrients to these vegetables have been identified and are being researched for other applications.

IMMUNE BOOSTER

Cruciferous vegetables, such as broccoli and kale, have been shown to not only boost the immune system, but to actually suppress tumor cells.

Blueberries

Blueberries have become famous for their antioxidant power—they are packed with more antioxidants than any other fruit or vegetable. The antioxidants in blueberries are believed to not only improve immunity, but also decrease your risk of cardiovascular disease and cancer, improve your skin and mind, and fight many of the overall signs of aging. And because of blueberries' extremely high antioxidant activity, their effect on various diseases has been studied directly. Research has suggested that regular consumption of blueberries can reduce belly fat, improve blood sugar and cholesterol, and reduce risk of heart disease and cancer.

Blueberries contain high amounts of vitamin C, but that's not what gives the antioxidants their immune-boosting properties. Blueberries also contain phytochemicals known as anthocyanins that give blueberries their bluish hue. These anthocyanins have antioxidant activity, as well as direct immune-strengthening properties. In addition, just one small serving of blueberries has approximately 16 grams of fiber, nearly half of the U.S. RDA. The fiber in blueberries promotes colonic health and less sugar absorption and stimulates certain factors that promote helper T cell production.

Mushrooms

Mushrooms are a type of fungus. Like probiotics (see Chapter 12), they can stimulate the immune system in the colon to produce a stronger immune response throughout the body. Because of this, mushrooms have been known for some time to be potent immune boosters.

In addition, like many other immune boosters, mushrooms have been more recently shown to have cancer-suppressing activity. This repeated connection is not coincidental, knowing that a strong immune system can help suppress cancer cells.

There are hundreds of different species of mushrooms, and research has been performed to see if certain mushrooms have a stronger immune-boosting and anticancer effect. No definitive evidence has shown that certain mushrooms are better than others, though, so try to eat different types of mushrooms, rather than certain ones over others.

Sweet Potatoes

Like cruciferous vegetables, sweet potatoes are loaded with the potent antioxidants vitamins A and C. In addition, sweet potatoes have plenty of vitamin B_6 (pyridoxine) and fiber.

With regard to vitamin A specifically, a serving of sweet potatoes contains almost four times the U.S. RDA of vitamin A, and a small cup of mashed sweet potatoes contains almost eight times the U.S. RDA! This means sweet potatoes are an easy way to take large amounts of vitamin A and therefore the beta-carotenoids (one of the types of vitamin A) that enhance the cell-mediated and humoral active and adaptive immune responses.

IMMUNITY ALERT

In addition to being loaded with the antioxidant vitamin A, sweet potatoes have plenty of fiber to stimulate the immunity of your gut.

Sweet potatoes contain plenty of other nutrients as well. In fact, they have been shown to contain so many nutrients that entire books have been written purely on the benefit of sweet potatoes.

Pomegranates

Pomegranates—in addition to being extremely tasty—offer a broad exposure to most antioxidants and are known to have anti-inflammatory benefits. The nutrients included in pomegranates are as follows:

- Copper
- Iron
- Selenium
- Zinc
- Vitamin A
- Vitamins B_1, B_2, B_3, B_5, B_6, and B_9

By having a broad exposure to different nutrients instead of containing an extraordinary amount of any individual nutrient, pomegranates help ensure against certain vitamin deficiencies that can contribute to immune deficiencies—it's almost like a fruit multivitamin!

Grains

The largest component of most diets is grains. While there has recently been concern about consuming too many carbohydrates from grains, leading to increases in insulin and fat storage, your body can benefit from low-glycemic, high-fiber grains that provide a steady source of energy and promote colonic health.

Bran

While bran may have once been known as a food for your grand-parents, it's getting more and more attention from everyone for its many positive nutritional qualities. Bran is loaded with fiber, which promotes colonic health and stimulates the immune system while decreasing the amount of excess carbohydrates that get absorbed and insulin and cortisol spikes. This smoothing of hormonal spikes decreases pro-inflammatory fat storage or immune-suppressing cortisol due to the lack of a sudden blood sugar drop that comes with simple carbohydrates like sweets.

Bran goes beyond just its fiber and carbohydrate content, though. Bran also contains free radical–binding antioxidants in the form of *polyphenols* (if you recall, free radicals contribute to inflammation and hurt immunity). The amount of these antioxidants varies by type of bran—for example, the black and sumac varieties of sorghum bran have a higher concentration than even blueberries, the highest antioxidant-containing produce!

DEFINITION

Polyphenols are substances with multiple phenols, or carbon rings. Phenols are what give grains their biologic antioxidant activity.

The beneficial antioxidant polyphenols in both of these types of bran are not only higher than blueberries, but have 5 to 10 times the antioxidants per serving of blueberries. Because of this, bran has actually been studied in mice and shown to reduce inflammation. Not all brans have been shown to have this beneficial effect on the immune system though, so if buying bran, aim for black or sumac sorghum bran.

Oats

Oats are an excellent source of low-glycemic carbohydrates and fiber and are also packed with many other immune-enhancing nutrients that benefit immune and overall health. Oats contain a specific type of fiber known as beta-glucan, which has been shown to have numerous health benefits.

Beta-glucan fiber has long been known to reduce bad cholesterol levels and decrease the risk of cardiovascular disease, which is why oat bran has long been promoted for heart health. More recently, beta-glucan fiber has also been shown to boost immunity by not only aiding the most predominant immune cells—neutrophils—to travel to infections, but also assist them in eradicating the offender.

IMMUNITY ALERT

Beta-glucan fiber has been shown to have heart and immune benefits even beyond the known health benefits of fiber.

Oat bran's cardiovascular and immune benefits are not just in the fiber, but also in other nutrients. Oat bran is loaded with antioxidants that offer the many health and immune benefits already described, including binding damaging free radicals. In addition, a single small serving of oat bran contains nearly 20 percent of the U.S. RDA of selenium and zinc. As discussed in Chapter 10, selenium has both antioxidant and immune-boosting properties, and zinc has been shown to reduce the severity and possibly the incidence of the common cold.

Lentils

In addition to being a high-fiber and high-protein food, lentils are packed with a broad array of immune-strengthening nutrients, leading to an overall boost in immune health.

Specifically, lentils are good sources of vitamins B_3, B_5, and B_6, as well as folate, iron, selenium, and zinc. The B vitamins support metabolism and prevent any B-vitamin deficiency (see Chapter 10) that would hamper the immune system. The folate and iron support cellular production, including immune cells and oxygen-carrying red blood cells, which maintain organ health and oxygenation that staves off infections. As with oat bran, selenium and zinc offer antioxidant benefits that strengthen the immune system as well. Between all of these nutrients, lentils provide a broad and comprehensive immune boost.

In addition, lentils are a strong source of protein compared to most grains. Lentils contain nearly all essential amino acids, but to make lentils a complete protein, you can pair it with a complementary amino acid source, such as rice. You can also allow them to sprout, which will change their nutritional components to create a complete protein source.

IMMUNE BOOSTER

Lentils are already a great source of immune-boosting nutrients and fiber. To make them a complete protein source as well, eat sprouted lentils from the market, or grow them yourself by simply letting lentils sit in water for a few days.

Wheat Germ

Though "germ" may have a negative connotation, wheat germ is an incredibly powerful immune booster. Like lentils, wheat germ contains a broad array of immune-boosting nutrients and fiber and has a high amount of protein. Wheat germ also provides healthy unsaturated fatty acids, which are essential in immune and cardiovascular health.

Wheat germ contains significant amounts of most B vitamins and nearly half the U.S. RDA of iron and copper. Even more impressive, a single serving of wheat germ contains approximately 100 percent of the U.S. RDA of zinc and selenium! The high concentrations of all of these nutrients provide a huge immune boost.

Furthermore, like lentils, wheat germ has a high amount of protein, though it is not a complete protein. You can complete this by combining it with nuts or seeds (discussed in the next section). Lastly, wheat germ contains a high amount of healthy fatty acids that promote good cholesterol, reduce bad cholesterol, and are anti-inflammatory, improving immune and overall health.

Dairy, Meat, and Nuts

Dairy, meat, and nuts are high-protein foods. They supply the essential nutrients for muscle and other tissues. Certain sources of protein are far healthier than others, and many contain far more immune-boosting nutrients. By optimizing your sources of protein, you can improve your immunity and your overall health.

Yogurt and Kefir

Yogurt and kefir, a milk fermented with kefir grains, contain many immune-boosting nutrients and are more easily tolerated in lactose-intolerant people. The most important of these nutrients is live, active cultures, or *probiotics.*

 DEFINITION

Probiotics are substances that contain and stimulate the growth of healthy microorganisms, which may confer a health benefit to the host.

Probiotics are live, healthy bacteria that have been shown to improve digestion, produce nutrients, and significantly improve the body's immune system (read more about probiotics in Chapter 12).

The amount of probiotics in yogurt and kefir can vary significantly. Unfortunately, most of the time the amount of probiotics is not listed, unlike in supplements. Regardless, it is worth looking at the labels. These strains and their benefits will be discussed in more detail in Chapter 12, but a simple rule is to look for as many different strains as possible. Strains that include *Bifidobacterium* and *Lactobacillus* are the best, as they have been shown to have the greatest beneficial effect on immunity.

The effect of yogurt on the immune system has been studied, and while all yogurt was shown to reduce the incidence of upper-respiratory infections, yogurt with live, active cultures has the greatest effect.

Salmon

Despite being a great source of protein, salmon has extremely high concentrations of another valuable nutrient: *omega-3 fatty acids.* Salmon is the most easily accessible and consumed fish high in omega-3 fatty acids, but the other types high in it include smelt, shad, anchovies, and sardines. Farmed fish such as farmed salmon may not be as beneficial.

DEFINITION

Omega-3 fatty acids are unsaturated fatty acids with a specific chemical structure that can promote health. Certain fish, eggs, and flaxseeds are common sources for omega-3 fatty acids. You can also get your omega-3s by taking fish oil supplements.

Omega-3 fatty acids are considered the healthiest fats in existence. Initial interest in omega-3s stemmed from studying the Eskimo population who, despite being heavier, had very low rates of cardiovascular disease. It is believed that this is due to a diet high in wild fish, especially wild salmon.

Since then, omega-3s have been extensively studied and shown to strengthen the immune system as well as reduce the risks of many chronic diseases, ranging from cardiovascular disease, to cancer, to dementia, to even depression. It is believed some of this effect may be due to a known anti-inflammatory effect of omega-3 fatty acids.

The beneficial effects of omega-3s may have to do with the fact that historically most societies lived near the sea and consumed high amounts of wild fish, so people may have evolved to do so. If you cannot tolerate fish such as salmon, consider an omega-3 supplement. Unfortunately, omega-3s do not appear to be something that everyone should consume higher amounts of, because even though on average they appear to have beneficial effects, these benefits are not necessarily seen in everyone, and some people develop a worsening of certain inflammatory and cholesterol biomarkers. Consider tracking your biomarkers or even your blood levels of omega-3 fatty acids through your doctor or a wellness service to see if adding salmon to your diet would help boost your immunity.

IMMUNITY ALERT

Many scientists feel that society's worsening cardiovascular health, weaker immunity, and increased prevalence of chronic diseases have to do with our decreased consumption of omega-3 fatty acids.

Brazil Nuts and Almonds

Fish are not the only great source of protein and healthy fats. Many types of nuts have it all—protein, healthy fats, and even fiber—giving you broad and balanced exposure to every type of macronutrient. What make certain nuts extra special are their micronutrients.

Brazil nuts and almonds contain many different types of nutrients, many of which are helpful for immunity. They supply iron, which supports the development of oxygen-carrying red blood cells, and are a rich source of zinc, which can decrease the severity and incidence of viruses such as the cold. Brazil nuts and almonds also contain a broad array of free radical–binding antioxidants. What makes Brazil nuts and almonds truly special is their amount of selenium—just one small Brazil nut or a couple almonds supplies more than the U.S. RDA of selenium!

As discussed in Chapter 10, selenium deficiency is something many people unknowingly have that has been associated with immune deficiency. To correct this, many foods are fortified with selenium; however, fortified supplements may have decreased "bioavailability," or percentage that can get actively absorbed. The selenium in Brazil nuts is known to have high absorption rates, and research has actually shown that just two Brazil nuts a day significantly increases selenium levels in the blood.

> **IMMUNE BOOSTER**
>
> Just a few nuts a day will supply fiber, protein, some healthy fats, and many antioxidants, including your daily needs of selenium.

The downsides with eating nuts are they have a relatively high concentration of saturated fat compared to many immune-supporting foods, and certain enzymes in these nuts may partially interfere with antioxidant absorption. Therefore, while nuts may be part of a balanced immune diet, they are best to enjoy in moderation.

Pumpkin Seeds

Like nuts, pumpkin seeds are an excellent source of protein and healthy fats. Though they don't contain the fiber of nuts, they do have the broad array of antioxidants present in nuts, as well as other immune enhancers.

Pumpkin seeds contain extremely high amounts of zinc. Just one small serving of pumpkin seeds contains nearly half the U.S. RDA of zinc, which can help stave off and reduce the duration and severity of colds.

Furthermore, pumpkin seeds contain other constituents called *phytosterols*, or cholesterol-like compounds found in plants, that are believed to support immunity. In addition, they have been clearly shown to reduce cholesterol levels and may even reduce your risk of cancer.

Drinks and Spices

Though it's great to have so many foods that are good for your immune system, you can only eat so much. Thankfully, food is not the only great sources of immune-strengthening nutrients. Many drinks and spices are packed with substances that can boost your immunity. By combining immunity foods with these drinks and spices, you can ensure a well-balanced, immune-boosting diet.

Green Tea

Despite being one of the most widely drunk beverages in the world for millennia, green tea has become popular in the United States only in the last few decades; however, its popularity has grown dramatically as word of the many of the benefits it offers has spread. Green tea is loaded with various nutrients that have been claimed to treat many different diseases and promote many different aspects of health. Generally, when so many claims are made about a food or drink, you should be skeptical. But in the case of green tea, there may be some validity.

In addition to containing many different antioxidants, over a half dozen other nutrients found in green tea have been shown to have health benefits. Certain benefits of these nutrients—which include catechins, alkylamines, and several others—involve boosting your immunity, providing cancer-fighting properties, reducing cardiovascular disease, and improving your complexion.

Furthermore, green tea has long been consumed by many societies with a relatively low amount of chronic disease and high longevity. Of course, other factors exist, but green tea has long been used for medicinal purposes in these societies. While many traditional folk remedies have fallen out of favor with experience or research testing, green tea has stood the test of time.

Garlic

Like green tea, garlic is loaded with different types of immune-boosting nutrients. While garlic may not actually keep a vampire away, it has been shown to fight various infections. Garlic includes key nutrients such as allicine, ajoene, and thiosulfinates, in addition to plenty of antioxidants. These have been shown to help fight bacteria, fungi, and even viruses.

> **IMMUNE BOOSTER**
>
> You can use raw garlic juice as a home remedy for minor fungal or bacterial infections of the skin, such as a skin yeast infection or inflammation from a cut. Raw garlic juice on the skin has been shown to be as or more effective than antibacterial and antifungal creams!

Furthermore, like zinc, some evidence exists that garlic, when taken at the start of the cold, will reduce the overall duration of it. However, this benefit in garlic has not been studied nearly as well as in zinc and therefore remains inconclusive.

Studies suggest that garlic may reduce the risk of cardiovascular disease, high blood pressure, and even different types of cancer. One study showed immune activity improvement with garlic consumption to be especially prominent in those with cancer.

Honey

Perhaps no sweetener or spice has more nutrients than honey. Honey has over 5,000 enzymes, several dozen vitamins and minerals, and a full complement of amino acids. In addition to having many of the antioxidants of other immune-boosting foods, honey has been shown to have antibacterial properties. Like raw garlic juice, raw honey can treat topical wounds and burns with very good effectiveness.

In laboratory studies, honey even at various low concentrations has been shown to stimulate many immune factors and immune cells. So between its antioxidant, antibacterial, and immune-boosting properties, honey is a veritable triple threat against infections.

> **IMMUNE BOOSTER**
>
> Instead of the usual sweeteners like sugar or artificial sweeteners, consider using immune-boosting honey to sweeten drinks and desserts.

Turmeric

Turmeric, a spice often used in curries, has been used for hundreds of years in traditional Chinese and Ayurvedic medicine for many different conditions. It is an excellent source of antioxidants and potentially has anti-inflammatory effects.

Because of this longtime use, turmeric has been formally studied and shown to reduce certain cancer indicators and the severity of symptoms in those who have cancer. The mechanism for this reduction in symptoms had not been completely understood, and only recently has a proposed mechanism for these effects come to light.

The key ingredient of turmeric is curcumin, which gives turmeric its color and is believed to be responsible for turmeric's anti-inflammatory and anticancer effects. In laboratory studies, turmeric has actually been shown to be poisonous to cancer cells. Curcumin appears to do this by making cell membranes more orderly and strengthening them. By curcumin improving cell membrane functioning, the cells become more resistant to infections and cancer, making it a potent immune booster.

The Least You Need to Know

- Foods can be your first source of many natural immune-boosting nutrients.
- Fruits and vegetables are full of antioxidants and phytochemicals that improve the function of your immune system.
- Low-glycemic, high-fiber grains provide a steady source of energy and promote colonic health.
- Dairy, meat, and nuts are high-protein foods that supply the essential nutrients for muscle and other tissues.
- Drinks and spices—such as green tea, garlic, honey, and turmeric—are packed with substances that can boost your immunity.

Supplementing Your Immunity

In This Chapter

- Probiotics and their immune-boosting power
- Immune-strengthening herbal supplements
- Do-it-yourself remedies to boost immunity

Foods are not the only thing you can ingest that will improve your immunity. Many supplements can strengthen your immunity, and many more claim to. This chapter focuses on the most common supplements that claim to or do boost your immunity and offers some tips on how to decide what works best for you.

Because you have so many options, you may feel overwhelmed. Don't try to consume all of these supplements; instead, think about which ones can realistically be incorporated into your life as you learn more about them.

Probiotics

Probiotics are the best immune-boosting supplements on the market. They have, by far, the most research evidence showing a definitive link between them and improvement in the immune system. It is also fairly well understood how probiotics improve the immune system.

But not all probiotics are created equal. Probiotics come in different types, quantities, and other varieties, all of which have different levels of effectiveness. By understanding probiotics, you can choose the most effective probiotic supplement for you.

Probiotics and the Immune System

Many people don't understand what probiotics are. Probiotics are essentially the opposite of antibiotics—they are supplements of bacteria.

It may be difficult to understand why you should consider taking a supplement of bacteria: *Aren't bacteria bad for me? Am I not supposed to go to significant lengths to make sure bacteria stay out of my food and to avoid bacterial infections?*

If you recall from Chapter 1, bacteria can be either bad or healthy. Healthy bacteria are actually quite vital to your health because they produce vitamins, stimulate your immunity, aid in digestion, and perform many other vital functions. Antibiotics are indiscriminate and kill both good and bad bacteria, making them harmful to your immunity.

Probiotics were initially developed to deal with this issue and replace the good bacteria killed by antibiotics. It wasn't long before it was discovered that probiotics were also helpful in people not taking antibiotics, which is why they have exploded in production and use over the last two decades.

Many theories abound about why added bacteria may be helpful in those not taking bacteria-suppressing medication. One theory is that most people are likely "bacteria deficient," and probiotics help correct that deficiency. People are exposed to far less bacteria than they were originally evolved to and are more sanitary because of hand washing and food sterilization and pasteurization. While this is beneficial for the population, like antibiotics, such processes eliminate people's exposure to healthy bacteria as well.

The most accepted notion of how probiotics support the immune system is that they stimulate the extensive amount of lymphoid tissue in the gut. This immune tissue, when exposed to bacteria, produces more cells and antibodies that then get circulated throughout the body and strengthen the overall immune system.

This immune system improvement is not just theoretical. Plenty of research has shown that those taking probiotics have higher levels of various immune markers and a decrease in a variety of illnesses.

Probiotics have other proven benefits as well. Because they aid in digestion, many people take them to regulate digestion and bowel issues. Probiotics reduce the incidence of diarrhea, C. diff infections, and yeast infections associated with antibiotic use. In other words, when it comes to boosting immunity, the first supplement you should consider is probiotics.

Probiotics also appear to improve people's cholesterol profile, reduce the risk of heart disease, lower blood sugar, and lower the risk of diabetes. But because probiotics have only become more popular over the last two decades, these other benefits have yet to be extensively studied and proven.

Types of Probiotics

Many different types of healthy bacteria exist, and certain healthy bacteria confer more benefits than others. Because probiotics are still fairly new, it is not fully understood which specific bacteria confer the most benefit; however, some general beneficial bacteria have been identified.

One of the most common and well-studied probiotics is *Lactobacillus*. Like most probiotics, *Lactobacillus* is found in the gut in varying amounts. Because *Lactobacillus* is one of the most studied and proven probiotics, it is also the most common probiotic supplement.

 IMMUNITY ALERT

More than 50 different strains of *Lactobacillus* exist, but it is not known which strains confer the most benefit.

Lactobacillus earned its name because the bacteria convert the sugar lactose to lactic acid. Therefore, *Lactobacillus* can be helpful for digesting lactose in those with lactose intolerance. The lactic acid *Lactobacillus* generates is also thought to suppress bad bacteria, another benefit of probiotics.

The other most commonly studied and supplemented probiotic is *Bifidobacterium*. *Bifidobacterium* is the most common bacteria already existing in the colon, comprising approximately 90 percent of colonic bacteria, so it makes sense to supplement with bacteria that are already indigenous to our gut.

Other common types of probiotics include:

- *Saccharomyces boulardii*—This is the only yeast probiotic. Like the more common probiotics, this can help prevent the overgrowth of C. diff and any other diarrhea associated with antibiotics.
- *Streptococcus thermophilus*—Like *Lactobacillus*, it contains the digestive enzyme for lactose and, therefore, can potentially be used as an aid for lactose intolerance.
- *Leuconostoc*—This can help ferment vegetables, improving digestion of certain produce.
- *Enterococcus faecium*—Commonly found in stool, certain forms can be virulent, while most are innocuous.

With so many different types of probiotics, how can you know which to take? While the answer is not clear, you can gain some insight into what might be the most effective by considering the likely mechanism of probiotics.

Because probiotics likely work by stimulating lymphoid tissue in our gut, the logical way to do this the most is by exposing the tissue to different types of probiotics. And because immune factors are so diverse, different bacteria will likely stimulate the production of different immune cells and antibodies. Therefore, you can get the widest production from having the greatest breadth of exposure.

So when searching for a probiotic supplement, look for one that contains many different types of probiotics, including one or ideally multiple strains of *Lactobacillus* and *Bifidobacterium* as well as other probiotics. The more varied the probiotic, the more diversely your immune system will benefit.

Amount of Probiotics

Like any other medicine or supplement, dose matters when taking probiotics. Fortunately, doses of probiotics are measured quite precisely by colony-forming units (CFUs) . You can think of CFUs the same way you think of milligrams or IUs in other medicines and supplements.

Probiotic supplements vary sharply in the number of CFUs. Some are only in the thousands, while others are in the tens of billions. Like any other supplement or medication, higher doses are more effective, though at some point a dose can likely be too high or harmful. Unfortunately, no clear answer can be given for the optimal dosage, but a harmful dose has yet to be found.

Though higher-dose probiotics exist, the highest dose widely and affordably available in nearly any drug or grocery store is 10 billion CFUs. This is also the dose recommended by many microbiologists, based on the limited best evidence for probiotics so far. Therefore, aim to take approximately 10 billion CFUs of probiotics per day. Though 10 billion sounds like a lot, a CFU is so small that 10 billion can easily fit in one small capsule.

IMMUNITY ALERT

Though approximately 10 billion CFUs of diverse probiotics per day is recommended, scientists have yet to find a dose high enough to be harmful.

To ensure you're getting an adequate dose of probiotics, refrigerate them to maintain the highest potency. Bacteria, like any other live ingestible, need refrigeration to preserve them. Therefore, even if the supplement doesn't indicate a need for refrigeration, do so in order to make sure your probiotics don't lose their potency as quickly.

Unfortunately, most probiotic supplements aren't refrigerated on the display shelves. Therefore, when examining a probiotic supplement, see if you can identify a date of manufacture. The more recent the production, the less time the bacteria have had to decompose and the higher the effective dose will be.

Finally, as with any supplement, different manufacturers might produce items of varying quality. No clear, objective source is available to say with certainty what company makes the best probiotics (though each manufacturer will of course tell you it's them). As probiotics grow in popularity, there will likely be more independent testing and rating of supplements and companies, so keep an eye out for these sorts of studies to get objective evidence of who makes the best probiotics.

So in short, aim to consume at least 10 billion CFUs per day of diverse probiotic strains, keep your supplies refrigerated, and try to use the best strains possible. Doing this will benefit your immunity and digestion and possibly provide many other benefits.

Herbal Supplements

Though probiotics are an excellent way to boost your immunity, many other supplements can strengthen your immunity, too. The evidence for the following options is not as strong as with probiotics, but they are popular immune supplements regardless. Ultimately, whether to try these supplements will be your decision; the following sections will give you a basic overview of each type and offer advice on how to decide what is best.

Acai Berry

The acai berry is an approximately 1-inch-long, reddish fruit native to Central and South America. Acai berry has become an incredibly popular supplement over the last decade, and the essence of the berry has been put into many over-the-counter supplements and added to foods, drinks, and even cosmetics.

Its purported benefits range from anti-aging, to weight loss, to reducing the risk of heart disease, to even improving complexion.

Acai berry is thought to be so effective because it has extremely high concentrations of antioxidants, anthocyanins, and flavonoids (see Chapter 10).

In general, antioxidants and anthocyanins are in higher concentrations in fruits, especially berries. Acai berries appear to have the highest concentration of these nutrients, which is why they are thought to be so much more potent.

While limited evidence is available showing that acai berry is actually effective, a part of this limitation—as with probiotics and other supplements—is their relative novelty. There hasn't been enough time to study all the possible benefits of acai berry in great detail.

IMMUNITY ALERT

Generally, when a supplement like acai berry is suggested to have many benefits, you should be skeptical. However, that doesn't mean such suggestions should be dismissed—just that there should be enough convincing evidence even if the theory is sound. While most supplements have limited evidence as to their effectiveness, this doesn't mean they can't boost your immunity.

However, we do know that on a physiological level, the substances in acai berry (such as antioxidants) are potentially helpful in many diseases related to aging; therefore, acai berry is believed to have a similar benefit. If you choose to take an acai berry supplement, it is important to know if the potent ingredients have been preserved in processing. To do this, look at the label of the supplement and see if it shows the concentration and amount of antioxidants or other beneficial substances. Acai berry supplements with higher amounts of these ingredients will be more effective than those with lower amounts.

Elderberry

Elderberry is another supplement that has become increasingly popular over the last decade. Like acai berry, elderberry is full of antioxidants and phytonutrients, with similar theoretical benefits, and is thought to have many health benefits beyond the immune system.

A small amount of research evidence suggests elderberry can reduce the severity of flu symptoms. In addition, some research has shown increased production of cytokines, an immune mediator, when elderberry is ingested. This research is limited and has no definitive conclusions, but because of these findings, elderberry is thought to be a potent immune booster.

Because of these potential benefits, elderberry has been used to fight viruses and atypical flus. Elderberry is even used by people with immune deficiencies, such as HIV, to boost their immunity. And some people use elderberry to potentially reduce inflammation (see Chapter 4 for more on inflammation and its connection to immunity). In fact, elderberry appears to be such a powerful immune booster that some people believe those who need to take medications to suppress their immunity should avoid elderberry, though there is no evidence to support this suggestion.

Though research on all the benefits of elderberry is still in its infancy, it has been used and studied enough to say that this supplement doesn't seem to have harmful effects. However, like any other supplement, medication, or nutrient, there's a possibility it could be dangerous at high levels. At the typically consumed levels, though, the biggest harm these supplements might do is cost you more money for no greater immune benefit. Check out the last section in this chapter for tips on how to evaluate various supplements like elderberry to gauge their effectiveness.

Echinacea

Though acai berry and elderberry have surged in popularity in recent years, echinacea has been one of the most popular immune supplements for more than a half century. In fact, even prior to that, echinacea was a traditional remedy used by native people of North America.

Echinacea is a group of nine species of flowering plants found in North America. However, the actual echinacea herb is only present in part of the plant. So, like with any other processing, make sure an echinacea supplement is actually the herbal extract and not just a portion of the plant.

Echinacea is probably one of the best-researched immune supplements, with dozens of studies from prestigious universities that have analyzed echinacea's effects on immune function. Unfortunately, despite all this research, there are no clear answers. Some *meta-analyses* show evidence that taking echinacea supplements can reduce the incidence of the common cold by up to a half! Other studies have shown reduced duration and severity of various viruses due to ingestion of echinacea supplements.

DEFINITION

Meta-analysis refers to the combined analysis of various individual studies.

Unfortunately, other studies have failed to repeatedly substantiate these findings, meaning the jury is still out. With all the historical use and some evidence, what is true of echinacea is similar to other immune supplements—it may be helpful. It is also possible certain supplements help some people and not others, as people are all different genetically and may respond differently to various supplements.

Echinacea has been shown to have interactions with various medications, so if you are considering taking echinacea, just like with any other supplements, make sure to discuss it with your doctor. Echinacea is also known to decrease the breakdown of caffeine, making its effects last longer in the body. This can cause jitteriness in people who ingest both caffeine and echinacea and, because caffeine is an immune suppressor, decrease the effectiveness of the supplement. So if you do take echinacea, make sure to avoid caffeine.

Echinacea can be taken in many different forms, including tablet or liquid, and the dose varies markedly, depending on what the form is. Despite this variation in dosages, echinacea supplements are designed to supply the effective doses for its specific form, but make sure to look at the label to make sure the amount of echinacea in a supplement you are considering is comparable to most other echinacea supplements. Most common dosages are approximately 900 mg of the powdered form or 6 to 9 ml of the liquid form.

Ginseng

Like echinacea, ginseng has been used for centuries by various cultures to help battle illness. Ginseng has also been proposed to have many other potential benefits—from reducing heart disease, to reducing lung diseases, to aiding concentration—but these benefits have yet to be proven in research.

Ginseng is an herb that comes in two main forms: American ginseng and Asian (or Korean) ginseng. Though American ginseng is more commonly ingested (to the point where it has been overharvested and is in more limited supply), it is believed that Asian ginseng is considered potentially more stimulating to your immunity.

Most ginseng supplements have a concentration of 4 to 5 percent of ginsenosides, the active ingredient of ginseng. A dose of 100 mg to 200 mg has been most studied and is what's recommended for this concentration. Of course, ginseng supplements with different concentrations of ginsenosides will have different recommended dosages.

Like other supplements, ginseng has many possible medication interactions, so discuss it with your physician first before you take ginseng. Similar to echinacea, ginseng may decrease the metabolism of caffeine, which could cause increased hyperactivity and potentially suppress your immune system. Ginseng is also known to decrease the effectiveness of blood-thinning medications like Coumadin (Warfarin), so either avoid ginseng or have your Coumadin levels checked more frequently if you decide to take it.

Do-It-Yourself Remedies

Though supplements have increased in popularity over recent years, the most popular immune boosters are the ones you can do at home. Certain foods are commonly used to decrease the duration and severity of the illness during times of sickness. This section focuses on some of these popular home remedies. (You can find other food immune boosters in Chapters 10 and 11.)

Chicken Soup

Chicken soup is the most traditional home remedy for illness. Because chicken soup can be made in thousands of different ways, no specific chemical in chicken soup can be pointed to as having infection-fighting properties. Rather, it is the basic ingredients in chicken soup that may offer some benefit when you are ill.

When you are ill, you often have an irritated throat and stomach or just have less of an appetite in general. Because of this, you tend to consume less food and liquid. Unfortunately, this can be the worst thing you do when you are ill.

Your body's energy needs often increase when you are sick, because infectious organisms or the fever your body produces in response to an infection can increase your metabolism. If you remember from Chapter 9, when you don't consume enough calories to maintain an adequate blood sugar, your body responds by releasing cortisol to raise your blood sugar. Cortisol is a potent immune suppressant, so having elevated cortisol can increase the duration and severity of your illness.

Furthermore, your body needs a moderate amount of fluids to function well. These needs increase when you're sick, for several reasons. Infections not only increase your energy needs, but your fluid needs as well. Fevers, by increasing your body's heat, greatly accelerate your body's consumption of fluids. In respiratory infections, increased breathing, especially through the mouth, will cause fluid evaporation and loss through your respiratory system. Not consuming enough fluids to keep up with these increased needs can lead to dehydration. Dehydration will only increase the fatigue and malaise associated with illness, and the decreased circulation of fluids can hamper immune circulation and the passage of harmful byproducts of infection.

IMMUNE BOOSTER

Though fevers can be uncomfortable, they actually improve immune function. Many people believe that fevers are treated because they are harmful to the body, but they are generally treated purely for comfort.

Chicken soup helps rectify some of your food and liquid needs. Taking small, warm spoonfuls of chicken soup is often easier on your throat and stomach. And because it's mostly liquid, chicken soup can help you stay hydrated. A combination of chicken and other ingredients, such as vegetables and noodles, supplies you with necessary carbohydrates and protein for energy and isn't laden with unhelpful amounts of saturated fat.

So while chicken soup may not contain a specific powerful supplement, because of its main ingredients of liquid broth, lean protein, and complex carbohydrates, chicken soup can be a great food when you are ill.

Phytonutrients

Phytonutrients and phytochemicals are just terms to describe various nutrients or chemicals found in plants. For example, herbal supplements such as acai berry, elderberry, ginger, and echinacea would be considered phytonutrients, as would any chemical in a fruit or vegetable.

When sick, some people increase their consumption of fruits and vegetables to combat their illness. Because produce has a higher concentration of water than most foods, they are a good way to help replace your fluid needs and supply lean carbohydrates for energy. Fruits and vegetables also potentially have other nutrients that can battle illness, including vitamins, antioxidants, and natural chemicals that can have immune-boosting or anti-inflammatory effects.

In general, it is always a good idea to increase your consumption of fruits and vegetables. Doing so can support our immune system to help stave off infection and—when you're dealing with an infection—supply hydration, energy, and other immune-boosting effects.

Airborne

Airborne has been a popular over-the-counter cold remedy since its inception in the 1990s. Airborne claims to reduce the duration and severity of the common cold when taken at the first sign of it.

Airborne contains many immune-boosting vitamins, minerals, and supplements, including the following:

- Amino acids (the building blocks of protein)
- Echinacea
- Magnesium
- Selenium
- Vitamin A
- Vitamin B$_2$
- Vitamin C
- Vitamin E
- Zinc

Airborne also contains a few other substances, such as artificial sweeteners.

The effectiveness of Airborne has never been studied, leading to lawsuits and attention from the Federal Trade Commission because of their claims. Most of the various ingredients in Airborne have not been shown to reduce the severity of illness once you're already sick, with the exception of zinc, but the doses of zinc in Airborne are approximately 10 percent of the recommended dose. In addition, zinc is supposed to be most bioactive when used as a lozenge under the tongue instead of swallowed in a pill like Airborne.

To date, no scientific studies have clearly demonstrated that Airborne acts as a general immune booster to decrease the chance of getting sick. Many of the ingredients in Airborne are antioxidants or have other activity, so they may potentially be effective, though this has yet to be definitively answered.

Emergen-C

Emergen-C has become very popular over the last decade, and like Airborne, it contains a mix of vitamins and minerals, though this mix varies by type.

> **IMMUNITY ALERT**
>
> Airborne and Emergen-C have no definite research supporting their claims to increase immunity or decrease the extent of illness.

Emergen-C varies in flavors and its exact ingredient profile, though the predominant ingredients are consistent throughout its products. Emergen-C is a powder that is put into liquid, where it dissolves and fizzes. In theory, being a dissolvable powder can lead to faster absorption of ingredients, though whether this makes an actual difference in its effectiveness is unknown. Emergen-C also markets itself as an energy product, in addition to helping prevent and fight off infections.

The following are the predominant ingredients in Emergen-C and their approximate amounts as a percent of the U.S. Recommended Daily Allowance (RDA):

- Vitamin C: 1500 percent U.S. RDA
- Vitamin B_6: 500 percent U.S. RDA
- Vitamin B_{12}: 400 percent U.S. RDA

Though these amounts sound like a lot, they have been studied and shown to not cause any harm. They have also not been clearly shown to have any benefit for preventing or fighting infections.

There are many other vitamins and minerals in Emergen-C in much lower amounts (less than 50 percent U.S. RDA), including vitamin B_2, niacin, magnesium, chromium, and zinc. As discussed with Airborne, though certain minerals like zinc may have some infection-fighting benefits, this is typically in higher amounts and in lozenge form.

No scientific studies have clearly demonstrated an immune-boosting effect from taking Emergen-C. Though clear benefits have yet to be established in research, you can surmise from the ingredients that it's unlikely to cause any harm unless you're unfortunate enough to have an adverse reaction to it.

IMMUNITY ALERT

By trying a supplement, you may be able to better understand what benefits your body and decide what works for you. But such decisions should be made carefully, and even before you try one, you should make sure you've researched it.

How to Decide What Works

With so many immunity superfoods, vitamins, minerals, and supplements, how do you decide what to take? You want to take what's most effective, and you certainly don't want to spend money on immune boosters that don't boost your immune system!

While deciding between the nearly limitless options of what to take to boost your immune system, you don't have to reinvent the wheel. Like you, millions of people are interested in what strengthens immunity, including many researchers. Tens of thousands of research studies exist on how various things you can ingest affect your immune system, many of which are cited throughout this book. However, you don't have to be limited to the research we've provided. When considering a certain food, vitamin, mineral, or supplement, go online and do research of your own. With most potentially immune-strengthening options, you'll find at least some research to suggest whether that option is or isn't effective. Look for true scientific studies rather than just manufacturer or unofficial claims.

Even if a lot of formal research has not been done, hundreds of thousands of people have tried the exact same option you're considering. What has their experience been like? Though these reports may be more anecdotal, if you put together many user experiences, you can have a better understanding of the general effect individuals have had with a supplement. Of course, this is not as conclusive as academic research.

What may benefit someone else may not necessarily have the same effect on you, as people are genetically, environmentally, and behaviorally unique. Since people's bodies vary, specific vitamins and minerals might benefit some, while other vitamins and minerals might be more effective for others.

You can analyze the effect on yourself in several ways. One way is to try something you are considering and pay attention to your health and illness. While this is perhaps the best method, it can certainly take some time to determine whether you are getting sick less and whether the infections are less severe.

Another more recently available option is actually measuring your immunity. Various biomarkers can give you a better understanding of your immune functioning. You can ask your doctor to order these tests in order to learn more about the impact on your immune system. Unfortunately, most doctors are reticent to do such testing when you aren't actively sick with a suspected immune condition.

Over the last few years, certain services have been developed that connect you with providers who can facilitate such testing. One that one of the authors is personally involved with (though receiving no financial benefit for mentioning) is WellnessFX. This service combines diagnostic testing with provider consultations to give you insight into the various biomarkers that are tested. You can learn more about this type of testing in more detail in the next chapter.

The Least You Need to Know

- Of all immune supplements, probiotics have the most evidence supporting them. Probiotics should be taken at a dose of at least 10 billion CFUs per day.

- Many more immune supplements have mixed data concerning their effectiveness, though some benefits have been shown in taking them.

- The key to a good home remedy is that it supplies adequate hydration and energy for your body's increased needs.

- Paying attention to academic research, your extent of sickness, and personal biomarkers while on immune supplements is the best way for you to gauge their effectiveness.

Steps Toward a Healthier Life

4

To help you get started with your new, immune-boosting health plan, this part contains 25 recipes for healthy, delicious breakfasts, snacks, and desserts. The nutrition information is listed with each recipe, the ingredients used in the recipes are immunity superfoods, and the preparations are easy in skill level. So the recipes are not only good for you, they're simple to make, too!

Perhaps the hardest part of adopting a new health plan is making a long-term commitment to changing your habits—and keeping up that commitment. This part helps you with that hurdle by sharing some strategies to help you make changes and stick to them.

Immune-Boosting Meals

In This Chapter

- Immune-boosting and nutrient-rich whole foods
- Hearty breakfasts
- Savory lunches and dinners

The cornerstone of an immune-boosting diet is using fresh, unprocessed foods when you prepare your meals. In addition, certain foods pack more nutritional value per calorie than others.

When you're pressed for time, it's easy to reach for that can of soup or a frozen entrée. But if you want to boost your immunity, you really need to eat what makes you healthy. Try to avoid foods that require you to read labels. Opt instead to purchase fresh fruits and vegetables from the produce department and meat and seafood from the refrigerated sections of the grocery store.

The recipes in this chapter use flavorful ingredients that also happen to be fresh, "whole" foods that are known to boost your immunity by lowering inflammation and providing plenty of antioxidants and omega-3 fatty acids.

Just as important as seeing the nutritional and immune-boosting value of these recipes is seeing just how easy cooking hearty meals can be. Start with these recipes, and then choose some of your favorite ingredients and experiment with your diet. Above all, have fun!

Kim Ross, MS, RD, CDN, of Kim Ross Nutrition (kimrossnutrition. com) provided the recipes for this chapter and Chapter 14. Kim has been involved in nutrition education for over 10 years and specializes in corporate wellness seminars and holistic nutrition workshops in the New York area. The recipes she provides in these chapters are designed to boost immunity and support good overall health.

Breakfasts

Veggie Egg Scramble

The subtle onionlike flavor of leeks combines with shiitake mushrooms, broccoli, and red bell pepper to create a flavorful egg scramble rich in vitamin C.

Yield:	Prep time:	Cook time:	Serving size:
2 egg scrambles	5 to 8 minutes	5 to 8 minutes	1 egg scramble

Each serving has:		
223 calories	103 calories from fat	11.5 g total fat
4.2 g saturated fat	0 g trans fat	333 mg cholesterol
231 mg sodium	19.6 g total carbohydrates	4.7 g dietary fiber
4.2 g sugar	14 g protein	25% vitamin A
67% vitamin C	12% calcium	36% iron

4 large organic eggs	½ cup chopped shiitake mushrooms
1 tsp. ghee	½ cup chopped broccoli
1 chopped leek	½ cup chopped red bell pepper

1. In a medium mixing bowl, whip eggs.

2. Heat a medium, nonstick frying pan over medium-high heat. Melt ghee in the pan.

3. Add leek, shiitake mushrooms, broccoli, and red bell pepper, and sauté until tender.

4. Add eggs to the pan, and scramble as desired.

5. Place egg scramble on a plate, and serve.

IMMUNE BOOSTER

Ghee, or clarified butter, contains saturated fat but is healthier overall than traditional fats, such as lard and margarine. You can buy ghee in most health-food stores or in the health-food aisle of most grocery stores. You can also find ghee at most Indian markets. Look for it on the shelf—ghee does not need to be refrigerated.

Steel-Cut Oatmeal with Kiwi, Banana, and Blueberries

Steel-cut oats are heartier than quick oats, and when combined with kiwi, banana, and blueberries, they offer a flavorful and nutritious power breakfast.

Yield:	Prep time:	Cook time:	Serving size:
3 bowls	5 minutes	20 to 30 minutes	1 bowl

Each serving has:		
169 calories	19 calories from fat	2.1 g total fat
0 g saturated fat	0 g trans fat	0 mg cholesterol
10 mg sodium	35 g total carbohydrates	5.3 g dietary fiber
9.8 g sugar	4.5 g protein	1% vitamin A
49% vitamin C	4% calcium	8% iron

3 cups water	½ cup organic blueberries
1 cup steel-cut organic oats	1 peeled and sliced ripe banana
1 sliced kiwi	½ tsp. cinnamon

1. In a large saucepan, bring water to a boil.

2. Stir in steel-cut organic oats. Bring to a rolling boil, then lower heat to medium-low.

3. Simmer oats for 20 to 30 minutes, stirring occasionally.

4. Place oatmeal in medium bowls and add kiwi, blueberries, and banana.

5. Sprinkle with cinnamon and serve.

IMMUNE BOOSTER

Oatmeal is known for its role in maintaining healthy cholesterol levels. If high LDL (bad) cholesterol is something you struggle with, add some oatmeal to your diet. Steel-cut oats are especially hearty, making for a power breakfast or even a good light lunch.

Salmon and Cucumber Sandwich

Smoked salmon and cucumber on sprouted wheat bread create a protein-packed sandwich with a fresh flavor.

Yield:	Prep time:	Serving size:
1 sandwich	5 minutes	1 sandwich

Each serving has:		
203 calories	10 calories from fat	1.2 g total fat
0 g saturated fat	0 g trans fat	0 mg cholesterol
344 mg sodium	43.6 g total carbohydrates	6.8 g dietary fiber
8.5 g sugar	9 g protein	3% vitamin A
7% vitamin C	3% calcium	15% iron

2 slices Ezekiel flax sprouted whole-grain bread	¼ tsp. dried dill
2 slices (3 oz.) smoked wild nova salmon or wild canned salmon	½ sliced cucumber

1. Toast whole-grain bread in a toaster oven or regular oven until golden brown. Remove from the oven and place toasted bread on a plate.

2. Add smoked wild nova salmon to each bread slice. Sprinkle dill on top of salmon.

3. Top with cucumber slices and serve open-faced.

Fruit-and-Yogurt Smoothie

Mango, peaches, and blueberries deliver refreshing flavor in this tried-and-true smoothie.

Yield:	Prep time:	Serving size:
2 smoothies	5 minutes	1 smoothie

Each serving has:		
180 calories	17 calories from fat	1.9 g total fat
.9 g saturated fat	0 g trans fat	28 mg cholesterol
92 mg sodium	20.3 g total carbohydrates	3 g dietary fiber
15.9 g sugar	13.9 g protein	11% vitamin A
27% vitamin C	13% calcium	3% iron

½ cup plain organic low-fat yogurt	½ cup frozen peaches
½ cup plain organic low-fat *kefir*	½ cup frozen blueberries
½ cup frozen mango	1 scoop (1 heaping TB.) whey protein powder
6 ice cubes	1 TB. flaxseeds

1. In a blender, add yogurt, kefir, and mango and pulse until chopped.

2. Add 3 ice cubes and peaches and pulse until blended.

3. Add remaining 3 ice cubes, blueberries, whey protein powder, and flaxseeds and pulse until blended.

4. Blend until creamy smooth.

5. Pour into glasses and serve.

DEFINITION

Kefir is a very healthy, yogurtlike dairy drink that contains live colonies of microorganisms. The probiotic- and immune-boosting benefits of kefir surpass even those of live cultured yogurt.

Gluten-Free Walnut-Flax Banana Muffins

Quinoa flour and flaxseeds pump up the nutrients while the bananas, maple syrup, and cinnamon create an aromatic flavor in these delicious muffins.

Yield:	Prep time:	Cook time:	Serving size:
12 muffins	15 minutes	25 to 30 minutes	1 muffin

Each serving has:		
225 calories	94 calories from fat	10.4 g total fat
2.9 g saturated fat	0 g trans fat	37 mg cholesterol
244 mg sodium	27.7 g total carbohydrates	2.4 g dietary fiber
10.7 g sugar	6.5 g protein	2% vitamin A
2% vitamin C	4% calcium	4% iron

2 cups organic quinoa flour	3 TB. organic butter
1 cup chopped walnuts	2 large organic eggs
2 TB. flaxseeds	1 cup organic milk
1½ tsp. baking soda	½ cup maple syrup
1 tsp. cinnamon	1 peeled and smashed ripe banana
¼ tsp. sea salt	

1. Preheat an oven to 375°F.

2. In a medium bowl, mix quinoa flour, walnuts, flaxseeds, baking soda, cinnamon, and sea salt. Set aside.

3. In a saucepan over low heat, melt butter. Set aside.

4. In a large bowl, beat eggs. Add milk, most of melted butter, maple syrup, and smashed banana.

5. Add combined dry ingredients and mix slowly with handheld blender until blended.

6. Pour mixture evenly into prebuttered muffin tins.

7. Bake for about 25 minutes until muffins are slightly browned on top. If you'd like, you can poke a toothpick in the center and make sure it comes out clean and free of batter.

8. Cool for 10 minutes. Serve warm or at room temperature.

IMMUNE BOOSTER

Quinoa is a whole grain that offers high-quality protein, fiber, and a range of vitamins and minerals. You can find organic quinoa flour in the health-food section of most grocery stores.

Lunches and Dinners

Kim's Chicken Soup

Flavorful herbs make this hearty chicken soup a tasty part of any immune-boosting meal plan.

Yield:	Prep time:	Cook time:	Serving size:
4 bowls	15 minutes	2 hours	1 bowl

Each serving has:		
187 calories	32 calories from fat	3 g total fat
3 g saturated fat	0 g trans fat	45 mg cholesterol
332 mg sodium	28 g total carbohydrates	4.2 g dietary fiber
2.2 g sugar	13 g protein	76% vitamin A
17% vitamin C	11% calcium	23% iron

1 yellow medium onion	½ cup chopped fresh parsley
3 large carrots	½ cup chopped fresh dill
3 large stalks celery	½ cup chopped fresh thyme
4 garlic cloves	1 TB. whole black peppercorns
3 *leeks*	1 tsp. ground white pepper
8 cups water	1 TB. kosher sea salt
1 organic chicken or chicken pieces	

1. Rinse, peel, and cut yellow onion, carrots, celery, garlic, and leeks into bite-size chunks. Set aside.

2. Fill a large pot with water and add chicken. Cover and bring to a boil.

3. Add onion, carrots, celery, garlic cloves, leeks, parsley, dill, thyme, black peppercorns, white pepper, and kosher sea salt and cover.

4. Simmer for 2 hours or until chicken is opaque and soft and soup is clear to pale yellow.

5. Take chicken out of soup, remove skin and bones, and cut meat into bite-size pieces.

6. Return chicken meat back to soup.

7. Remove from heat to cool. Ladle soup into bowls and serve.

DEFINITION

Leeks are a mild-tasting member of the onion family. The long cylinder of bundled leaf sheaths—the white and pale green part of the plant—is the edible part. The dark-green leaves and rooted bottom can be discarded.

Lentil Soup

Celery, carrots, and onions add texture to this savory lentil soup.

Yield:	Prep time:	Cook time:	Serving size:
4 bowls	15 minutes	8 to 10 hours	1 bowl

Each serving has:		
227 calories	43 calories from fat	4.8 g total fat
.9 g saturated fat	0 g trans fat	0 mg cholesterol
6 mg sodium	34.5 g total carbohydrates	17.3 g dietary fiber
1.1 g sugar	13.1 g protein	5% vitamin A
11% vitamin C	11% calcium	33% iron

1 cup dry lentils, rinsed	4 garlic cloves, chopped
7 cups water	3 bay leaves
1 (2.5-oz.) pkt. miso soup mix	1 TB. dried oregano
⅔ cup chopped celery	1 TB. extra-virgin olive oil
⅔ cup chopped carrots	1 TB. red wine vinegar
⅔ cup chopped onions	1 TB. ground black pepper
¼ cup crushed rosemary	

1. Place lentils, water, miso soup mix, celery, carrots, onions, rosemary, garlic, bay leaves, oregano, extra-virgin olive oil, red wine vinegar, and black pepper in a slow cooker.

2. Cook overnight, about 8 to 10 hours, in slow cooker on low heat.

3. Remove bay leaves, ladle into bowls, and serve.

Tangy Skirt Steak and Tomato-Spinach Salad

Tamari soy sauce, scallions, garlic, lime juice, and spices create a tangy marinade for the skirt steak in this hearty dinner recipe. This flavor is balanced by the freshness of the tomato-spinach salad.

Yield:	Prep time:	Cook time:	Serving size:
2 steaks plus salad	1 hour 30 minutes	10 minutes	1 steak plus ½ salad

Each serving has:

530 calories	386 calories from fat	42.9 g total fat
8.2 g saturated fat	0 g trans fat	50 mg cholesterol
1,603 mg sodium	10 g total carbohydrates	2.9 g dietary fiber
2 g sugar	28.9 g protein	131% vitamin A
47% vitamin C	11% calcium	37% iron

⅓ cup extra-virgin olive oil	1 tsp. red pepper flakes
4 oz. (½ cup) gluten-free low-sodium tamari	1 tsp. cumin
½ cup lime juice	2 organic free-range lean skirt steaks
4 chopped scallions	4 cups chopped organic spinach
2 smashed garlic cloves	1 chopped organic tomato
1 TB. ground black pepper	¼ cup balsamic vinegar

1. In a medium bowl, mix 3 tablespoons extra-virgin olive oil, tamari, lime juice, scallions, garlic, black pepper, red pepper flakes, and cumin.

2. Pour mixture into a large zipper-lock bag. Add steaks, seal bag, and shake until steaks are covered with mixture.

3. Refrigerate in the bag and let marinate for 1 to 2 hours.

4. In a medium bowl, mix spinach and tomato. Set aside.

5. Remove steaks from the refrigerator and place in a sauté pan. Pour any leftover juice onto steaks.

6. Cook 5 minutes on medium-high heat on each side or until desired. Remove steaks and place on plates.

7. Drizzle balsamic vinegar and remaining extra-virgin olive oil onto tomato-spinach salad and mix.

8. Place tomato-spinach salad on top of steaks and serve.

Wasabi Salmon with Sweet Potato and Brussels Sprouts

Wasabi, tamari soy sauce, and honey create a complex flavor for the salmon in this recipe. The mellow sweet potato and bitter Brussels sprouts are perfect complements to the fish.

Yield:	Prep time:	Cook time:	Serving size:
2 salmon plus vegetables	15 minutes	35 minutes	1 salmon plus ⅓ vegetables

Each serving has:		
381 calories	167 calories from fat	18.6 g total fat
3.5 g saturated fat	0 g trans fat	56 mg cholesterol
1,502 mg sodium	31.5 g total carbohydrates	7.1 g dietary fiber
10.8 g sugar	23.1 g protein	360% vitamin A
164% vitamin C	7% calcium	16% iron

2 tsp. wasabi powder (dried Japanese horseradish)

1 tsp. toasted sesame oil

1 TB. gluten-free low-sodium tamari

1 tsp. raw honey

1 large sweet potato, sliced

10 organic Brussels sprouts

1 TB. extra-virgin olive oil

1 tsp. sea salt

6 oz. wild salmon filet

1. Preheat an oven to 450°F.

2. In a small bowl, mix wasabi powder, toasted sesame oil, tamari, and honey. Set aside.

3. Place sweet potato and Brussels sprouts in a roasting pan, drizzle with extra-virgin olive oil, and sprinkle with sea salt. Cover with aluminum foil and cook 35 minutes or until soft to the touch and bright in color.

4. Place salmon in a sauté pan and apply wasabi mixture with a cooking brush.

5. Cook salmon on medium-high heat for 4 minutes on each side or until desired.

6. Place salmon and roasted vegetables on plates and serve.

Lamb Chops and Ratatouille

Simple preparation with white pepper and sea salt allows the delicate flavor of the lamb chops to emerge in this recipe. The ratatouille combines flavorful and healthy vegetables and packs a whopping 105 percent of your daily recommended allowance of vitamin C.

Yield:	Prep time:	Cook time:	Serving size:
6 lamb chops plus ratatouille	25 minutes	35 minutes	1 lamb chop plus $\frac{1}{3}$ ratatouille

Each serving has:		
513 calories	266 calories from fat	29.6 g total fat
6.9 g saturated fat	0 g trans fat	153 mg cholesterol
528 mg sodium	11.3 g total carbohydrates	3.6 g dietary fiber
5.5 g sugar	50 g protein	36% vitamin A
105% vitamin C	6% calcium	29% iron

¼ cup extra-virgin olive oil	1 cup chopped organic tomatoes
½ cup chopped white onion	1 TB. chopped organic basil
3 chopped garlic cloves	1 TB. chopped organic parsley
1 cup eggplant	2 tsp. sea salt
1 cup chopped red bell pepper	2 tsp. white pepper
1 cup zucchini	6 lamb chops
1 TB. organic tomato paste	

Ratatouille:

1. Set a large sauté pan over medium heat and add extra-virgin olive oil.

2. Add onion and garlic and stir about 5 minutes.

3. Add eggplant and stir about 5 minutes.

4. Add red bell pepper, zucchini, and tomato paste and cook about 5 minutes.

5. Add tomatoes, basil, parsley, 1½ teaspoons sea salt, and 1½ teaspoons white pepper and cook for 5 more minutes.

6. Stir well to blend.

7. Let sit, covered, to keep warm.

Lamb chops:

1. Preheat an oven to 375°F.

2. Place lamb chops in a large, 4-quart glass baking dish.

3. Sprinkle remaining ½ teaspoon white pepper and remaining ½ teaspoon sea salt over lamb chops.

4. Cook in the oven, uncovered, for 8 minutes.

5. Turn and cook another 8 minutes, or until desired.

6. Remove from the oven when there's a deep brown crust on top and bottom. The inside can be cooked to your personal preference.

7. Place lamb chops on plates and serve with ratatouille.

Tofu Stir-Fry with Wild Rice

This tofu stir-fry is a classic dish made extra savory by the addition of wild rice.

Yield:	Prep time:	Cook time:	Serving size:
2 plates stir-fry plus rice	10 minutes	1 hour	1 plate stir-fry plus ½ rice

Each serving has:		
452 calories	132 calories from fat	14.6 g total fat
2.5 g saturated fat	0 g trans fat	0 mg cholesterol
336 mg sodium	65.7 g total carbohydrates	9.2 g dietary fiber
8.9 g sugar	20.7 g protein	109% vitamin A
149% vitamin C	24% calcium	35% iron

1 cup wild rice

2 cups organic free-range chicken broth

1 cup water

1 block (approximately 12 oz.) extra-firm organic tofu

¾ cup gluten-free reduced-sodium tamari

Juice of 1 lemon

2 TB. toasted sesame oil

½ cup chopped white medium onion

½ cup shredded carrots

½ cup fresh button mushrooms

½ cup chopped broccoli

½ cup chopped red bell pepper

1 cup snow peas

½ cup grated ginger

1 TB. red pepper flakes

Wild rice:

1. In a large saucepan, bring wild rice, chicken broth, and water to a boil on high heat.

2. Reduce heat to medium, cover, and simmer for 45 minutes.

3. Uncover and fluff wild rice. Keep on very low heat and stir occasionally.

Tofu:

1. Cut tofu into 1-inch cubes.

2. In a medium bowl, mix tamari, lemon juice, and tofu and marinate 1 hour. Set this aside while preparing vegetables.

3. Heat a large skillet. Add toasted sesame oil, onion carrots, button mushrooms, broccoli, red bell pepper, snow peas, ginger, and red pepper flakes and sauté over high heat for about 10 minutes. Vegetables should remain crunchy for best taste, so do not overcook.

4. Add tofu and marinade and stir 5 minutes.

5. Remove from heat and serve over wild rice.

IMMUNE BOOSTER

Most people don't know that wild rice is not technically rice at all. Rather, it's a gluten-free grain product derived from four different grasses that grow in North America and China. Wild rice is a nutrient-rich food that's high in protein and dietary fiber and low in fat. It's also a good source of certain minerals and B vitamins.

Four-Bean Chili

This vegetarian chili contains four types of beans and traditional chili spices, making for a hearty, savory meal on its own or served with a side salad.

Yield:	Prep time:	Cook time:	Serving size:
4 to 6 bowls	10 to 15 minutes	45 minutes	1 bowl

Each serving has:

444 calories	54 calories from fat	6 g total fat
1.3 g saturated fat	0 g trans fat	2 mg cholesterol
440 mg sodium	74.5 g total carbohydrates	19.6 g dietary fiber
7.6 g sugar	26.7 g protein	23% vitamin A
69% vitamin C	20% calcium	48% iron

1 cup canned organic kidney beans

1 cup canned organic white beans

1 cup canned organic black beans

1 cup canned organic garbanzo beans

1 cup crushed organic tomatoes

1 cup chopped organic yellow onion

1 cup chopped and seeded jalapeño pepper

1 cup chopped organic green bell pepper

1 cup chopped organic red bell pepper

½ cup organic vegetable broth

4 chopped garlic cloves

1 TB. extra-virgin olive oil

1 TB. chili powder

1 tsp. ground black pepper

1 tsp. salt

¼ cup organic chopped scallions

¼ cup shredded organic mozzarella cheese

1. Rinse and drain kidney beans, white beans, black beans, and garbanzo beans.

2. In a large pot, add kidney beans, white beans, black beans, garbanzo beans, tomatoes, yellow onion, jalapeño pepper, green bell pepper, red bell pepper, vegetable broth, garlic, extra-virgin olive oil, chili powder, black pepper, and salt.

3. Partially cover pot and simmer 45 minutes, stirring often.

4. Remove chili from heat and place into bowls.

5. Top with scallions and mozzarella cheese and serve.

IMMUNITY ALERT

Beans of all sorts provide the fiber you need to promote strong heart and gastrointestinal health. Stay away from canned baked beans, though, which are loaded with sugar and (sometimes) unnecessary fats.

Seafood Stew

Fennel and saffron add a unique twist to this protein-packed seafood stew. Mussels, sea bass, wild salmon, and baby clams combine to create a complex texture and varied flavor.

Yield:	Prep time:	Cook time:	Serving size:
2 bowls	2 minutes	about 30 minutes	1 bowl

Each serving has:		
282 calories	101 calories from fat	11.3 g total fat
1.7 g saturated fat	0 g trans fat	73 mg cholesterol
591 mg sodium	16.6 g total carbohydrates	2.7 g dietary fiber
4.5 g sugar	29.9 g protein	12% vitamin A
41% vitamin C	7% calcium	13% iron

1 TB. extra-virgin olive oil	1 cup organic chicken broth
6 garlic cloves	2 oz. mussels
1 cup fennel chopped	2 oz. sea bass, cut into chunks
½ yellow onion, chopped	2 oz. wild salmon, cut into chunks
1 organic tomato, chopped	2 oz. baby clams
¼ tsp. ground black pepper	2 oz. medium shrimp, peeled
1 TB. saffron	

1. In a large saucepan, add extra-virgin olive oil, garlic, fennel, and yellow onion.

2. Stir over medium heat until garlic, fennel, and onion are softened, about 5 to 8 minutes.

3. Add tomato, black pepper, and saffron and stir about 5 minutes.

4. Add chicken broth and bring to boil.

5. Reduce to a simmer and add mussels, sea bass, wild salmon, baby clams, and shrimp.

6. Simmer until seafood is opaque, about 3 minutes.

7. Place stew in bowls and serve.

IMMUNE BOOSTER

Seafood provides lean protein and is loaded with immune-boosting omega-3 fatty acids. Look especially for "steaklike" fish, such as tuna, swordfish, tuna, and sea bass.

Hearty Kale-Sardine Salad

The strong flavor of protein-rich sardines is mellowed by the complementary flavors of kale, almonds, and edamame in this hearty salad.

Yield:	Prep time:	Serving size:
1 salad	10 minutes	½ salad

Each serving has:		
426 calories	254 calories from fat	28.3 g total fat
3.7 g saturated fat	0 g trans fat	64 mg cholesterol
568 mg sodium	22.2 g total carbohydrates	7.6 g dietary fiber
2.7 g sugar	24.8 g protein	218% vitamin A
168% vitamin C	40% calcium	38% iron

2 cups kale	¼ cup sliced almonds
¼ cup fresh lemon juice	1 cup edamame, shelled
½ tsp. sea salt	1 (5-oz.) can wild sardines packed in water
3 TB. extra-virgin olive oil	
½ tsp. ground black pepper	

1. Soften kale by kneading it between your hands or on a cutting board with a sprinkle of lemon juice and a pinch of sea salt to soften and wilt it.

2. In a large bowl, mix kale, extra-virgin olive oil, remaining lemon juice, black pepper, and remaining sea salt.

3. Mix in almonds and edamame.

4. Split salad onto plates.

5. Drain wild sardines from can, place over salads, and serve.

Almond Butter and Cherry Sandwich

Sour cherries and ripe banana combined with almond butter create a flavorful pairing in this easy, nutritious sandwich.

Yield:	Prep time:	Serving size:
1 sandwich	5 minutes	1 sandwich

Each serving has:		
345 calories	85 calories from fat	9.4 g total fat
.9 g saturated fat	0 g trans fat	0 mg cholesterol
946 mg sodium	57.8 g total carbohydrates	11.1 g dietary fiber
19.2 g sugar	11.7 g protein	8% vitamin A
11% vitamin C	5% calcium	15% iron

2 slices seven-grain bread	6 organic sour or dried cherries
1 TB. organic almond butter	1 tsp. raw honey
¼ tsp. cinnamon	1 dill pickle
½ ripe sliced banana	

1. In a toaster oven, toast seven-grain bread until golden brown.

2. Spread almond butter onto toasted bread and sprinkle cinnamon on top.

3. Add banana slices and cherries and drizzle honey over fruit.

4. Close sandwich or eat open faced and serve with pickle.

IMMUNE BOOSTER

Although high in sodium, pickles are also high in probiotics. Eaten in moderation, they are a valuable addition to any immune-boosting diet.

Veggie-Filled Acorn Squash

This dish is a real treat if you like fresh, sweet food. Acorn squash and *jicama* are naturally sweet and nutritious. Celery and yellow pepper add crunch, while avocado and tomatoes add freshness.

Yield:	Prep time:	Cook time:	Serving size:
1 squash	10 minutes	45 minutes	½ to 1 squash

Each serving has:		
195 calories	6 calories from fat	.7 g total fat
0 g saturated fat	0 g trans fat	0 mg cholesterol
65 mg sodium	49.6 g total carbohydrates	8.3 g dietary fiber
3.1 g sugar	4.5 g protein	49% vitamin A
98% vitamin C	17% calcium	19% iron

1 medium acorn squash	½ cup celery, chopped
½ yellow pepper, chopped	½ avocado, chopped
½ cup cherry tomatoes	Salt and ground black pepper
½ cup jicama, chopped	(optional)

1. Preheat an oven to 450°F.

2. Cover acorn squash with aluminum foil and place on a baking sheet. Cook 45 minutes, or until squash is soft inside. (You can check with a knife for doneness.)

3. Remove acorn squash from oven, cut in half, and remove seeds. (Caution: squash will be hot.) Let cool.

4. In a medium bowl, mix together yellow pepper, cherry tomatoes, jicama, and celery.

5. Scoop vegetable mixture into center of squash.

6. Season with salt and black pepper (if using) and serve.

DEFINITION

Jicama is a root vegetable that resembles a turnip in appearance. It has a sweet flavor that lends well to fresh vegetable dishes. Jicama is a good source of vitamin C.

Healthy Snacks and Desserts

In This Chapter

- The importance of healthy snacking on your immune system
- Immune-boosting snacks
- Nutritious desserts

Who doesn't enjoy having a little snack during the day or a tasty dessert after dinner? Part of eating well is, well ... eating.

In fact, eating between meals is a healthy thing to do. Going too long without food between meals is destructive to your immune health because it causes your cortisol levels to rise, which in turn causes inflammation. Snacking on healthy, immune-boosting foods keeps your cortisol levels in check, which helps control inflammation and promotes strong immunity.

And so you can please your sweet tooth while still eating healthy, we've also included desserts, which you should treat as an end-of-day snack. They are easy to make and fun to eat.

Bon appétit!

Snacks

White Bean Dip and Carrots

Garlic and basil add a Mediterranean flavor to this white bean dip. Serve with organic baby carrots to get the most nutritional punch from this healthy snack.

Yield:	Prep time:	Serving size:
1 bowl dip plus carrots	8 to 10 minutes	¼ dip plus carrots

Each serving has:		
258 calories	68 calories from fat	7.6 g total fat
1.1 g saturated fat	0 g trans fat	0 mg cholesterol
166 mg sodium	37.5 g total carbohydrates	9.5 g dietary fiber
3.9 g sugar	12.7 g protein	192% vitamin A
21% vitamin C	15% calcium	32% iron

1 (15-oz.) can organic white beans or cannellini beans	2 TB. extra-virgin olive oil
2 cups organic baby carrots	2 TB. fresh lemon juice
3 garlic cloves	¼ tsp. white pepper
¼ cup fresh parsley	¼ tsp. sea salt
¼ cup fresh basil	2 cups organic baby carrots

1. In a food processor, place white beans, garlic, parsley, basil, extra-virgin olive oil, lemon juice, white pepper, and sea salt.

2. Pulse until mixture is chopped.

3. Purée until dip is soft. Scoop dip into a bowl.

4. Serve dip with baby carrots.

IMMUNE BOOSTER

Substituting raw vegetables for chips or crackers is an easy way to pump up the nutritional value of your snacks. Try having carrots, broccoli, cauliflower, bell peppers (any color), and grape or cherry tomatoes. Simple changes like this can reap big results.

Guacamole

Served with fresh vegetables or organic corn chips, this mellow guacamole is guaranteed to be a healthful crowd pleaser!

Yield:	Prep time:	Serving size:
1 bowl	10 to 15 minutes	½ bowl

Each serving has:

187 calories	134 calories from fat	14.9 g total fat
2.1 g saturated fat	0 g trans fat	0 mg cholesterol
248 mg sodium	15.4 g total carbohydrates	7.8 g dietary fiber
3.2 g sugar	3 g protein	15% vitamin A
54% vitamin C	2% calcium	5% iron

2 ripe avocados, peeled and scooped	½ cup chopped onion
	1 cup chopped organic cilantro
½ cup fresh lime juice	1 garlic clove, crushed
1 jalapeño pepper, chopped	½ tsp. sea salt
1 Roma tomato, diced	

1. In a medium bowl, place avocados.

2. Add lime juice and mix.

3. Add jalapeño pepper, Roma tomato, onion, cilantro, garlic, and sea salt and mix until evenly distributed and soft.

4. Serve with *crudités* (raw vegetables) or baked organic corn chips.

DEFINITION

Crudités are sliced or whole raw vegetables typically served with a variety of dips. Common crudités include carrots, bell peppers, broccoli, cauliflower, carrots, tomatoes, and asparagus.

Beet, Watermelon, and Spinach Salad

With a surprising blend of Dijon mustard and sweet watermelon, this salad is sure to delight.

Yield:	Prep time:	Serving size:
1 salad	10 minutes	½ or 1 salad

Each serving has:

95 calories	29 calories from fat	3.2 g total fat
0 g saturated fat	0 g trans fat	0 mg cholesterol
90 mg sodium	15.9 g total carbohydrates	2.9 g dietary fiber
11.7 g sugar	3.2 g protein	66% vitamin A
30% vitamin C	6% calcium	10% iron

1 tsp. extra-virgin olive oil

1 tsp. Dijon mustard

1 tsp. basil

2 cups organic fresh baby spinach

1 cup watermelon, cut into cubes

1 cup beets, cut into cubes

1. In a small bowl, mix extra-virgin olive oil, Dijon mustard, and basil. Set aside.

2. In a large bowl, mix baby spinach, watermelon cubes, and beet cubes.

3. Add olive oil mix to salad, toss, and serve.

Kim's Trail Mix

Goji berries bring a unique flavor to this trail mix and, when combined with various nuts, seeds, and dried fruits, make this trail mix a tasty, immune-boosting superfood.

Yield:	Prep time:	Serving size:
1 bowl	3 to 5 minutes	$\frac{1}{5}$ bowl

Each serving has:

194 calories	103 calories from fat	11.4 g total fat
1.6 g saturated fat	0 g trans fat	0 mg cholesterol
4 mg sodium	20.5 g total carbohydrates	3.4 g dietary fiber
12.9 g sugar	6.1 g protein	28% vitamin A
4% vitamin C	6% calcium	17% iron

½ cup Brazil nuts	¼ cup dried figs
½ cup organic raw almonds	¼ cup goji berries
½ cup pumpkin seeds	¼ cup organic raisins

1. In a medium bowl, place Brazil nuts, almonds, figs, goji berries, and raisins.

2. Mix together and serve.

DEFINITION

Goji berries, also called *wolfberries,* are a bright orange-red berry native to Tibet and Mongolia. Like many berries, goji berries are packed with antioxidants, which are valuable, immune-boosting nutrients.

Desserts

Vanilla Ice Cream with Cherries and Pomegranates

This vanilla "ice cream" is made from healthy coconut milk. Tangy cherries and pomegranates provide the perfect complement to the sweetness of the ice cream.

Yield:	Prep time:	Serving size:
1 bowl	3 to 5 minutes	1 bowl

Each serving has:		
200 calories	27 calories from fat	4 g total fat
0 g saturated fat	0 g trans fat	0 mg cholesterol
55 mg sodium	30 g total carbohydrates	5 g dietary fiber
23 g sugar	1 g protein	1% vitamin A
3% vitamin C	0% calcium	3% iron

½ cup So Delicious brand dairy-free, no-sugar-added coconut milk ice cream in Vanilla Bean	2 TB. pomegranate seeds
	2 TB. cherries

1. In a small bowl, place vanilla ice cream.

2. Top with pomegranate seeds and cherries and serve.

IMMUNE BOOSTER

If you can't find the So Delicious brand, you can use Coconut Bliss brand or any other vanilla bean ice cream made with coconut milk.

Chocolate Almond Coconut Balls

Organic dark chocolate and creamy almond butter create a decadent treat when combined with almonds, coconut, and dried cranberries.

Yield:	Prep time:	Cook time:	Serving size:
12 balls	15 to 20 minutes	10 to 20 minutes	1 ball

Each serving has:		
198 calories	110 calories from fat	12.2 g total fat
4.9 g saturated fat	0 g trans fat	3 mg cholesterol
13 mg sodium	21.3 g total carbohydrates	1.9 g dietary fiber
16.8 g sugar	3.2 g protein	1% vitamin A
2% vitamin C	6% calcium	5% iron

7 oz. (2 large bars) organic dark chocolate

½ cup chopped almonds

½ cup almond butter

½ cup raw honey

1 cup shredded coconut

1 cup dried unsweetened cranberries

½ tsp. nutmeg

¼ tsp. vanilla extract

2 TB. water

1. In a medium mixing bowl, add almonds, almond butter, honey, coconut, cranberries, nutmeg, vanilla extract, and water.

2. Knead mixture in the bowl until ingredients are evenly distributed. Set aside.

3. Break dark chocolate into pieces for melting. Place wax paper on a cookie sheet.

4. In a double boiler over low heat, place chocolate.

5. Stir until chocolate melts and appears shiny and smooth.

6. Remove chocolate from heat and stir.

7. Take tablespoon-size pieces of nut mixture and sculpt into balls (the size of large gumballs).

8. Dip balls in liquid chocolate until completely covered and place on wax paper.

9. Place in the freezer for 1 hour. Remove and serve.

Mixed Berry Crumble

Raspberries, blueberries, and strawberries add fresh flavor while cashews and sunflower seeds pump up the crunch in this crumble.

Yield:	Prep time:	Cook time:	Serving size:
About 12 squares	15 to 20 minutes	35 minutes	1 square

Each serving has:

109 calories	53 calories from fat	5.9 g total fat
2.7 g saturated fat	0 g trans fat	10 mg cholesterol
28 mg sodium	14.5 g total carbohydrates	2.5 g dietary fiber
9.2 g sugar	1.4 g protein	2% vitamin A
9% vitamin C	1% calcium	3% iron

½ cup raspberries

½ cup blueberries

½ cup strawberries

¼ cup sunflower seeds

¼ tsp. vanilla extract

½ cup raw honey

½ cup gluten-free all-purpose flour (such as Bob's Red Mill)

¼ cup chopped cashews

¼ cup melted organic butter

1. Preheat an oven to 350°F.

2. In a medium mixing bowl, place raspberries, blueberries, strawberries, all but 1 teaspoon sunflower seeds, vanilla extract, and honey and gently stir.

3. Slowly add all-purpose flour to mixture and gently toss.

4. Place berry-flour mixture in a square 8×8 pan.

5. Sprinkle remaining 1 teaspoon sunflower seeds and cashews on top and drizzle butter.

6. Place the pan in the oven and bake about 35 minutes, until berries begin to bubble.

7. Remove and cool.

8. Cut into squares and serve.

Fruit Parfait

A fabulous summertime treat, this fruit parfait combines the tangy flavor of raspberries and blackberries with the sweet crunch of muesli mixed with honey and coconut.

Yield:	Prep time:	Serving size:
2 parfaits	5 minutes	1 parfait

Each serving has:

180 calories	30 calories from fat	3.4 g total fat
2.3 g saturated fat	0 g trans fat	10 mg cholesterol
115 mg sodium	23 g total carbohydrates	3.2 g dietary fiber
17.3 g sugar	11.1 g protein	3% vitamin A
20% vitamin C	31% calcium	3% iron

2 TB. sugar-free muesli (such as Familia Swiss Muesli No Added Sugar)	1 TB. shredded coconut
¼ tsp. vanilla extract	2 cups organic low-fat plain yogurt
1 tsp. raw honey	½ cup raspberries
	½ cup blackberries

1. In a medium bowl, mix muesli, vanilla extract, ½ teaspoon honey, and coconut.

2. Cover bottom of 2 tall glasses with muesli mixture.

3. Layer ½ of yogurt over muesli mixture and layer ½ of raspberries and ½ of blackberries over yogurt. Repeat with remaining yogurt, raspberries, and blackberries.

4. Drizzle remaining ½ teaspoon honey on top and serve.

Mint-Chocolate Pudding

Fresh mint and cocoa together create a decadent delight for your taste buds. Almond milk and agave add just the right amount of complexity to the flavor.

Yield:	Prep time:	Cook time:	Serving size:
4 bowls	20 to 25 minutes	30 minutes	1 bowl

Each serving has:

144 calories	32 calories from fat	3.6 g total fat
1.2 g saturated fat	0 g trans fat	0 mg cholesterol
198 mg sodium	29.6 g total carbohydrates	6.1 g dietary fiber
16.5 g sugar	5.5 g protein	14% vitamin A
3% vitamin C	19% calcium	21% iron

½ cup fresh mint leaves	2 cups almond milk
2 TB. water	1 tsp. vanilla extract
2 organic egg whites	⅓ cup agave
⅔ cup unsweetened cocoa powder	¼ tsp. salt
2 TB. cornstarch	

1. In a food processor, blend mint leaves and water. Set aside.

2. In a small bowl, beat egg whites gently. Set aside.

3. In a large bowl, mix cocoa powder, cornstarch, 1 cup almond milk, mint mixture, and vanilla extract and whisk until smooth. Set aside.

4. In a large saucepan, mix remaining 1 cup almond milk, agave, and salt.

5. Bring to a boil over high heat, whisking continuously. Remove from heat.

6. Whisk cocoa mixture into milk mixture.

7. Bring to a boil over medium-high heat for 2 to 3 minutes, whisking continuously. Remove from heat.

8. Slowly whisk 1 cup hot cocoa mixture into beaten egg whites.

9. Pour mixture back into the pan and cook over medium heat, whisking continuously. Do *not* let mixture boil. Remove from heat.

10. Pour into 4 serving bowls.

11. Cool to room temperature and cover.

12. Refrigerate for about 1 hour. Remove bowls from the refrigerator and serve.

Change Your Habits, Change Your Life

In This Chapter

- Committing to new, immune-boosting changes
- Monitoring your progress through tests and other checks
- Ways to stay motivated

In this book, you have learned many actions you can take to improve your immunity. You can adjust your diet, activity, sleep, stress, and so much more! In other words, you now know how to strengthen your immunity to help prevent various diseases. Knowing is just half the battle, though.

The biggest challenge is implementing these changes into your life. With so many changes you can make, it's difficult to incorporate as many of them as you can for as long as you can. This chapter offers tips on how you can best do that to make significant, lasting changes in your life.

Committing to Change

Commitment doesn't just come naturally. Nor does it come from knowing a habit is good for you; if a change just being good for you were enough, everyone would be successful in quitting smoking or losing excess weight.

To truly be successful, you have to be zealously committed to making changes. Fortunately, research has provided some answers for what contributes to commitment and lasting change.

IMMUNITY ALERT

Like any sustainable change, improving your immune system requires planning and not trying to do too much at once. Slow, steady progress is much more effective than a sudden, rapid change.

Contemplation

The first step in contemplation is called *precontemplation*. This refers to whatever has happened in your life that has driven you to decide to make changes. Go back to what motivated you to read this book. What made you want to boost your immunity? You may be plagued with infections or on medications that suppress your immune system, or maybe you witnessed someone you care about have serious infections in their older age.

Whatever your reasons, at some point you consciously started contemplating wanting to boost your immunity. You made the active decision to read this book and, by reading it, started contemplating the various changes you could make that would strengthen your immune system. Therefore, congratulations—you've taken the first step.

This contemplation stage is not over, though. You should now think about the earlier chapters and all the consequences of having a weakened immune system. People with a weakened immune system have an increased risk of various infections, many of which are debilitating and some of which are just dangerous. Infections have both short-term and long-term risks not only on you but on those around you. A weak immune system has even been associated with an increased risk of cancer. Just as in thinking about your initial motivations, use all these benefits to increase your determination to strengthen your immune system.

Making a Plan

Just knowing how to improve your immune system is clearly not enough to make an impact in your health—you have to act on your newfound knowledge. Acting is not as simple as just changing your activity, stress, diet, and all the other potential ways to improve your immune system the next day. Implementing many changes requires planning and using your determination to stick to that plan.

Generally, singular changes are the easiest to implement and sustain. You want to make a change and continue with that change until it becomes a sustainable part of your life, which can take days to weeks. With so many changes you might want to make now, it could take a very long time to incorporate all the changes you are hoping to if you do them one at a time. However, there are tricks to accelerating this process.

IMMUNITY ALERT

Trying to do everything at once is nearly a guaranteed way to fall short of your goals. Consider and execute what order you want to make change and when you wish to make those changes.

Though making one change at a time is good idea—and making multiple changes in your diet, activity, or other areas is harder to maintain and sustain—you could potentially make a single change in multiple aspects of your life that can impact the immune system. By doing this, you are essentially making several changes at a time but in different areas. For example, you can make one change in your activity (such as going for a lunchtime walk), one change in your stress level (like doing five minutes of morning meditation), one change in your diet (like lowering the amount of saturated fat in what you eat for dinner), and one change in a supplement (such as having a daily probiotic capsule).

The goal after each change is to continue practicing it until it goes from effort to practice to habit. Usually this requires one to three weeks. Therefore, you can plan your schedule ahead of time as to what changes you want to make in your life, estimate how long it will take for it to become a regular practice in your life, and then figure out when you can implement other changes. By making this plan, you can prepare for your changes to be successful and sustainable.

Preparation

At this point, you've decided what changes you wish to make and an approximate schedule of when and how you want to implement these changes. To be able to follow this plan, you need to have many resources in place to be able to execute your changes.

The following are some tips for being prepared to implement various changes:

- If you plan to meditate (see Chapter 8), set aside a time. If you intend for it to be in the morning, plan to set your alarm clock earlier to allow for the amount of time you'll need.

- If you plan to change aspects of your diet (see Chapter 9), stock the fridge with the foods you'll need and begin to part with the foods that may be more harmful to your immune system.

- If you plan to use supplements (see Chapter 12), obtain whatever ones you need (such as probiotics) for when you are ready to begin them. And, in addition to the information in this book, feel free to research supplements further.

- If you plan to increase your physical activity (see Chapter 7), decide how and when and make sure the time is set aside to do so. Also, make sure you have the right gear.

IMMUNE BOOSTER

There are many more aspects to preparing for change, but the key is to make sure you have the resources available for when you decide to implement that change—whether it's time, equipment, or food.

Implementation

You have made the plan and ensured that you have the resources to successfully implement your changes. But even though you may have the ability to make a change, changing habits can still be tough, because doing so requires effort.

When it becomes time to actually make the change, you want to once again step back and return to motivation. At various points during the day when you'll be practicing your new habit, you may encounter some internal resistance. When you do, remember that by decreasing stress, improving your diet, and increasing your physical activity, you'll not only significantly improve your immune system and decrease your risk of infection, you'll also improve many other aspects of your health, including your heart and brain. The only side effects of all these interventions will be improved energy and mood. Your changes will positively influence others, and by having a stronger immune system, you'll also have a positive effect on those around you.

Though implementing changes may be challenging at first, each day it'll become a little bit easier. Eventually, you'll become so used to your new habits that it actually takes effort to stop doing it. For example, if you get used to eating certain types of foods and have those foods around you, you'd need to make an effort to find and eat unhealthy foods. Or if you get used to exercising every morning, it would then be a change to not do so. Your goal should be to get your habits to a point that it would be more disconcerting to not practice immune-boosting activities than to practice them.

Monitoring Your Progress

You have now started to do more immune-boosting activities. You have learned how these activities boost your immune system from this book, and you may have even taken it upon yourself to do extra research. Other than knowing that what you're doing should be improving your immune system, how can you ensure that your immune-strengthening changes are actually having their intended effects?

Checking Your Health Inside and Out

Just a few decades ago, blood tests didn't even exist. But like many products, over time blood tests have become far more prevalent, cheaper, and better. Tens of thousands of blood tests can evaluate nearly any physiological process, including your immune system. Though there are thousands of tests that evaluate your immune system (some of which have been commented on in earlier chapters), there are four key blood tests you can do to monitor your health.

One test is *white blood cell count*. Remember, your white blood cells are your immune cells and include neutrophils, lymphocytes, macrophages, and several other types of cells. A typical white blood cell count counts each of these types of cells.

Your actual white blood cell count will vary for various reasons. For example, in types of stress, more white blood cells get released into the blood, increasing your white blood cell count. Therefore, the white blood cell count is not really useful for comparison if the number of cells is within the normal range. Where the white blood cell count is useful is in identifying a deficiency in the overall number of white blood cells or any of the specific type of cell lines.

The next test is *high-sensitivity C-reactive protein (hs-CRP)*, which is the best test that exists for inflammation. Inflammation is the body's response to many types of trauma, illness, and infection. A part of the inflammatory response is the release of many immune factors, which can act as a distraction for the immune system in fighting the usual infections and other offenders that your immune system staves off. The hs-CRP test detects one of these inflammatory mediators, the C-reactive protein, to measure the overall levels of inflammation.

While acute inflammation can occasionally be part of the body's normal healthy response, persistent, chronic inflammation is associated with many diseases, including cardiovascular disease, cancer, dementia, and many other diseases. By reducing your chronic inflammation, you reduce your risk of many of these diseases, as well as improve your immune system.

Another test is the *basic lipid panel*, which helps you monitor your risk of cardiovascular disease. The basic lipid panel includes your total cholesterol and breaks it down into bad cholesterol and good cholesterol. Bad cholesterol, otherwise known as low-density lipoprotein or LDL, has been shown to clog blood vessels that feed your major organs (including your brain and your heart) and contribute to your risk of a heart attack and stroke. Good cholesterol, otherwise known as high-density lipoprotein or HDL, on the other hand, carries plaque away from arteries and helps decrease your risk of a heart attack and stroke. Also measured on the basic lipid panel is triglycerides, a type of fat that like LDL cholesterol has also been shown to contribute to vessel clogging or atherosclerosis.

Generally, your cholesterol and triglyceride levels can be improved by getting more physical activity, eating less saturated fat, and committing to other actions recommended to strengthen your immunity (such as decreasing stress).

A fourth blood test you can use to evaluate your immune system is a test for your *globulins*. Globulins are the main type of immune proteins in the body, with one type of globulin—your gamma-globulins—being your body's antibodies. In other words, the globulin test checks the antibodies of your immune system.

As with the white blood cell count, this test is used best as a check for deficiency. Also similar to the white blood cell count, globulins can be broken down into individual types. In fact, the gamma-globulins can be broken down further into individual types of antibodies. Unlike the white blood cell count, though, where this breakdown is performed routinely as part of the test, tests for antibody deficiencies are only specifically performed when a deficiency is suspected. If you have low amounts of a specific type of antibody, you may be more susceptible to infections this type of antibody fights.

IMMUNE BOOSTER

You can check your internal health in many ways without making and waiting for multiple doctor appointments. Try an online service like WellnessFX (wellnessfx.com), which is designed to be easy and affordable by giving you the ability to access your results and speak to health professionals from home.

Through your physician or a wellness testing service, you can routinely check your biomarkers to monitor inflammation or any deficiencies in your immune system.

Monitoring Any Sickness

The most important measure of your progress is how you feel. Think about how often you develop some form of illness and the nature of the illness you develop. By comparing the frequency and severity of your illnesses before you started strengthening your immune system to after you began immune-boosting changes, you can better understand if the actions you're taking are having their intended effect.

To see what differences have been made by making changes to boost your immunity, ask yourself these basic questions:

- How often do you get viruses, such as colds? Three times a year? More or less?
- Do you typically get the flu every year?
- Do you often get other infections, such as stomach bugs?
- How often do you take antibiotics?
- How much do you miss work each year for sickness?
- Do you ever have to be hospitalized for illness? If so, how often?

By thinking about the prevalence of these in the past and monitoring their occurrence in the future, you can evaluate whether your immune-strengthening activities are having their intended effect of making you healthier.

Feeling the Other Effects

The great thing about many of the things you can do to improve your immune system is they only have positive side effects. These effects range from how you feel to the health of many systems of your body. Like your immune system, these feelings and other effects can be monitored.

Improving your diet, decreasing stress, and increasing your physical activity all should improve your energy and mood. You can keep track of these changes by asking yourself certain questions:

- Are you having an easier time focusing and getting more done?
- Do you feel less sluggish, with less desire to take naps?
- How do you feel about life in general? Do you enjoy activities more?

Most likely you will say *yes* to all these questions, and you can use this to motivate you further.

Staying Motivated

Once you have implemented changes to boost your immunity, you'll need to stay motivated to continue these changes. Fortunately, maintaining these changes is much easier than initially implementing them. If you can remember what motivated you to improve your immune system in the first place and recognize the positive effects the changes are having on your life, you should be very capable of continuing these sustainable activities in your life. The key is to recognize the improvements you are making in your life and the lives of those around you while forgiving yourself for any imperfections on your path.

IMMUNE BOOSTER

Often people fail to make sustainable changes because they revert back to old habits. Therefore, maintaining motivation is important until the change becomes the habit.

Forgiving Imperfection

No one is perfect, no matter how hard you try to be. Regardless of your level of effort, there will be days where you do something that is not optimal in boosting your immunity. This could be anything from not commencing an activity the day you intend despite your contemplation and planning, to deciding to take a day off from something you have progressively implemented in your life.

For example, you may miss exercising one day, or you may let stress get to you instead of taking time to relax. Alternatively, you may do certain activities that you've been avoiding that you know are detrimental to your immunity, such as eat an unhealthy meal or not get enough sleep.

It's okay! Again, no one is perfect. There's no question that you will not be able to do everything you can to boost your immunity. What is far more important is how you deal with the times you go off plan. The most important thing is not to let it stress you out—after all, stress hormones are immune suppressors. In other words, if you let it bother you too much, you will only compound the immune-harming effects.

On the other hand, don't let the desire to avoid stress take away from your motivation to continue your immune-strengthening behaviors. It's easy to let a little slip justify no longer doing the behavior because you feel you've fallen off the path. Remember, though, the path of boosting your immunity is a journey, not just a destination. The strength of your immune system is not majorly influenced by a single behavior on a single day; it's the sum of all your behaviors every day. Also, your immune system will be more affected by more recent behaviors, so regardless of what you did or didn't do yesterday, what you do today matters more. Again, don't use the fact that one day doesn't have too strong an effect as an excuse to skip practices, because it becomes easy to fall back into old habits.

Strive to be the best you can, but forgive yourself for not being perfect. You are only human, and just the fact that you have boosted your immunity and are working toward strengthening it even further is admirable. Instead of letting imperfection deter your path, be proud of your continued progress.

Recognizing Your Progress

Earlier, we discussed how you can track the changes you've made to make sure your interventions are effective. Even more important than tracking your progress is recognizing and enjoying it.

Many people lose a certain amount of productivity in their lives due to illness. You may have had less time for work, your family, or any other important aspects of your life. You may have been a *nidus* of infection, spreading illness to those around you. If you've found you are getting sick less, remember what it was like to get sick often and how, with your new immune-boosting activities, you're able to accomplish more. You may have more time for earning or success at work or to spend with your friends or family.

DEFINITION

A **nidus** is the point of origin for a disease, most commonly referenced as the starting point of an infection.

And don't just think about the short term—think about how you've likely added years to your life while reducing time and expenses devoted to treatment of illness. You not only decrease your risk of various diseases by decreasing infections, you also change the impact of these diseases through the new, healthier activities in your life. Being more active, decreasing stress, and improving your diet all have a profound effect on your risk of heart disease, cancer, diabetes, and many other chronic diseases.

Such significant changes are in your grasp, and as you make changes, think about the long-term effects and recognize the value you have already obtained. Essentially, by working to strengthen your immunity, you are not just boosting your immune system—you're boosting many aspects of your life.

IMMUNITY ALERT

Unlike many health interventions that can have significant negative side effects, the interventions in this book generally have only positive effects. Eating healthier, being more physically active, and reducing stress have all been shown to improve mood and increase energy. These only further improve your productivity and ability to do activities for work, family, and friends. In other words, you can not only add to your life span, you can also add to your quality of life.

Improving the Lives of Those Around You

By practicing many of the techniques in this book, you have not only boosted your immune system, reduced your risk of infectious illness or future chronic diseases, and improved your mood and energy. You have made the world around you a better place.

Most infectious illnesses are spread person-to-person. This pathway requires that each person along the path contract the infection. As discussed at many points in this book, improving your immunity decreases the duration and severity of illnesses and the chance of even being infected by an illness and your infectivity to others. In other words, by strengthening your immunity, you decrease the likelihood that you spread the infection to other people, starting with the people you spend most of your time around—your family and friends.

You also help those around you by being a positive influence. It is well known that people learn most of their behaviors from others around them, whether it's your family, friends, co-workers, or others. By improving your immunity and other aspects of your health and life, you can inspire others to do the same.

And by limiting your own sickness, you can reduce your disability due to infectious illness and other chronic diseases while increasing your mood, energy, and life span. All of this allows you to contribute more of your time and ability to the world, whether via your family, friends, work, or other forms of service. Regardless, the more time and energy you can offer, the better you can make things around you.

Ultimately, the greatest way you can change the world is by changing yourself, or put more simply by Gandhi, "Be the change you want to see in the world." The positive impact you have on your own immunity and overall health and productivity is a microcosm of a change that could be seen in the world. Though your changes may only make a small difference in the health of the world, if others make similar changes in aggregate, the difference could be quite significant.

IMMUNITY ALERT

Studies have shown that taking action to improve your own health improves the health behaviors of others around you and, to a lesser degree, the health behaviors of the people around those around you.

In other words, the small difference you make in your immunity—and your overall health and life—are the first step to not only making a positive impact in yourself, but also in the world around you and at large.

Congratulate Yourself!

Though the key to strengthening your immunity is a few basic techniques, boosting your immunity is by no means easy. Even with all the positive effects on not only your immunity but on your life and the lives of others, making these changes requires effort and dedication. A key aspect of staying motivated is congratulating yourself for what you have accomplished.

You can congratulate yourself in different ways. You can simply praise yourself verbally in your own mind, or you can actually reward yourself for your adjustment in behavior. Perhaps the reward will be a fun activity or a nice meal. With such a potential reward in place, you will have motivation and incentive to adhere to techniques that boost your immune system.

Plus, by improving your immunity and overall health, you have increased your productivity and time, so feel free to use some of that time to do what you enjoy—you've earned it! And when you do an occasional activity you enjoy, you'll reduce your stress further, conferring even more of a benefit to your immunity.

By completing this book, you've taken the first big step in improving your immunity, your health, and your life. Congratulations!

The Least You Need to Know

- You are much more likely to be successful with careful contemplation and planning.
- Strengthening your immune system doesn't just require knowledge—it demands taking action to implement the changes.
- With time, the effort you make to change your lifestyle will become habitual and a more natural part of your life.
- Perfection is impossible, so focus on continued progress and the benefits conferred to yourself and those around you.

active immune memory   The long-term type of immune memory acquired by having an infection and through vaccines.

acute inflammation   A short-term, healthy response of the body to injury, infection, and other stresses.

adaptive immune system   The part of the immune system that remembers what antigens the immune system has encountered in the past, facilitating a stronger immune response with subsequent exposure.

allergen   A normally harmless substance that induces an immune response or allergic reaction. Common allergens include dust, mold, pollen, pet dander, and certain foods.

allergic reaction   Inflammatory immune reactions caused when the immune system releases histamines and other substances in response to exposure to an allergen.

allergy   A sensitivity of the immune system to a substance that is normally harmless. *See also* allergen.

anaphylaxis   A medical emergency characterized by swelling of the tongue or throat, trouble breathing, and low blood pressure. It is caused by a severe allergy, usually to a food allergen.

antibody   A protein used by your immune system to launch a direct attack on the antigens in your bloodstream.

antigen   A foreign substance or pathogenic bacterial, viral, fungal, or parasitic organism that elicits an immune response.

antioxidant An element that binds free radicals—which are thought to contribute to the aging process—that are produced through oxidation reactions in the body.

asthma An immune response characterized by wheezing and breathlessness. Asthma is often associated with an allergic reaction, but it can also be caused by exercise sensitivity, infection, or exposure to cold air.

atherosclerosis The buildup of plaque in your blood vessels that obstructs blood and oxygen flow to vital organs. It's also referred to as "hardening of the arteries."

autoimmune disease A condition where the immune system is overactive and attacks the body itself. It usually targets particular organs, depending on the specific disease.

B cell An immune cell that works by releasing antibodies into the body.

bacterial infection An infection caused by bacteria, microorganisms that often live on or in the body. Most bacterial infections respond to antibiotics.

biomarkers A marker of biological process. In the case of inflammation, biomarkers are used to identify the presence and severity of inflammation in your body.

C-reactive protein (CRP) The primary indicator of inflammation in your body. The higher your CRP level, the greater the amount of inflammation you have. Your doctor can check your CRP level via a simple blood test.

cell-mediated immunity An immune response that fights antigens by using T cells rather than antibodies.

chronic inflammation Increased inflammation that occurs over an extended period of time, usually caused by autoimmune diseases and lifestyle choices (such as diet, obesity, and stress).

Clostridium difficile (C. diff)   A bacterial infection that causes gastrointestinal symptoms, such as stomach pain and diarrhea. C. diff infections respond to antibiotics.

crudité   A sliced or whole raw vegetable typically served with a variety of dips. Common crudités include carrots, bell peppers, broccoli, cauliflower, carrots, tomatoes, and asparagus.

eczema   An allergic reaction in the skin characterized by itchiness, red hives, or scaly plaques.

Escherichia coli (E. coli)   A bacteria normally present in the gut, specifically in the colon. The most dangerous form of E. coli is generally transmitted as a food-borne illness and can cause a serious gastrointestinal infection.

fungal infection   An infection caused by fungi or more complex forms of yeast. A fungal infection has the same basic symptoms as a yeast infection.

goji berry   Also known as a *wolfberry*, a bright orange-red berry native to Tibet and Mongolia. Like many berries, goji berries are packed with antioxidants, which are valuable, immune-boosting nutrients.

herd immunity   How a society develops a common immunity to certain diseases. Vaccinations can play a role in developing herd immunity.

high-density lipoprotein (HDL) cholesterol   A healthy or good form of cholesterol. You can increase your level of HDL cholesterol by eating foods rich in omega-3 fatty acids (such as salmon and tuna) or taking fish oil supplements.

humoral immunity   An immune response carried out by antibodies.

immune deficiency   When the immune system is weakened or completely crippled, increasing the risk of infection.

immunity   Resistance to infection that develops when the immune system recognizes antigens it encountered previously.

inflammation   When your tissues swell, often turning red and feeling warm to the touch. It is part of the immune response that occurs when tissue becomes damaged or infected. While short-term inflammation may be a useful part of the immune response, having increased inflammation over an extended period of time is considered unhealthy. *See also* acute inflammation *and* chronic inflammation.

innate immune system   The layer of the immune system that works at the cellular level to consume and destroy antigens.

jicama   A root vegetable that resembles a turnip in appearance. It has a sweet flavor that lends well to fresh vegetable dishes. Jicama is a good source of vitamin C.

kefir   A very healthy, yogurtlike dairy drink that contains live colonies of microorganisms. The probiotic- and immune-boosting benefits of kefir surpass even those of live cultured yogurt.

leeks   A mild-tasting member of the onion family. The long cylinder of bundled leaf sheaths—the white and pale green part of the plant—is the edible part. The dark-green leaves and rooted bottom can be discarded.

low-density lipoprotein (LDL) cholesterol   A bad form of cholesterol. LDL cholesterol transports fats and cholesterol to artery walls, damaging and clogging your arteries.

lymph node   A spherical, ball-like junction of lymph vessels. Lymph nodes contain an extremely high concentration of immune cells used to kill antigens that pass through them via the lymphatic fluid.

lymphatic system   A network of organs, nodes, and vessels with a high concentration of lymphoid tissue. The lymphatic system cleanses the blood and fights infection. *See also* lymphoid tissue.

lymphoid tissue   Tissue throughout the body that's full of immune factors. Lymphoid tissue is present in everything from the linings of mucosa, to condensed areas, to entire organs.

lymphoma   A tumor in a lymph node, as is seen in Hodgkin's and non-Hodgkin's lymphoma.

macronutrient   The carbohydrates, proteins, and fats that are the core of what people eat and that support energy and tissues.

memory cells   Specialized B cells and T cells that are the basis of immune memory, a key aspect of the adaptive immune system.

meta-analysis   The combined analysis of various individual studies.

methicillin-resistant Staphylococcus aureus (MRSA)   A bacterial infection that affects the skin and is resistant to common antibiotics.

micronutrients   All the other nutritional components, such as vitamins and minerals.

mucosal immune system   The part of the immune system that works to maintain the health of your mucous membranes. *See also* mucous membrane.

mucous membrane   The inner lining of your body that gets exposed to the outside environment. Mucous membranes are present in the digestive, respiratory, reproductive, and urinary tracts.

nidus   The point of origin for a disease, most commonly referenced as the starting point of an infection.

normal flora   Microorganisms that live on your skin and mucous membranes. Many are considered beneficial; others are considered to be antigens.

omega-3 fatty acids   Unsaturated fatty acids with a specific chemical structure that can promote health. Certain fish, eggs, and flaxseeds are common sources for omega-3 fatty acids. You can also get omega-3s by taking fish oil supplements.

opportunistic infection   An infection that doesn't normally pose a threat but becomes active when a person's immune system is weakened.

parasite   An organism that lives in or on another organism (its host) and benefits by deriving nutrients at the host's expense.

passive immune memory   A type of immune memory that lasts from a few days to several months. Passive immune memory can be found in infants, who share immunity from their mother.

phagocyte   A large, white cell that can engulf and digest antigens. Phagocytes include monocytes, macrophages, and neutrophils.

phytochemical   A chemical compound that occurs naturally in plants that may promote health.

polyphenol   A substance with multiple phenols, or carbon rings. Phenols are what give grains their biologic antioxidant activity.

probiotic   A substance that contains and stimulates the growth of healthy microorganisms, which may confer a health benefit to the host.

sensitization   When an antigen is administered to provoke an immune response. This way, the body has a stronger response the next time it sees the antigen and therefore is able to better deal with the exposure.

stroke   A blood clot or the rupture of a blood vessel that stops the flow of blood to the brain.

surface barrier   The body's first defense against antigens. The surface barrier includes the skin, the lining of the respiratory tract, and the stomach.

T cell   A type of white blood cell that regulates the immune system. *Helper T cells* recognize antigens and activate the appropriate immune cells to attack them, while *killer T cells* actually kill antigens.

vaccine   Medicine that protects against disease by mimicking an antigen and provoking a response from your immune system; this creates immune memory of the antigen so your body can better defend against the disease upon exposure. Vaccines are administered by injection, oral solution, or inhalant.

viral infection   An infection caused by a virus or pieces of genetic material that get inside healthy living cells and cause the cells to become sick. Viral infections do not respond to antibiotics.

yeast   A fungus that flourishes in warm, moist environments, such as certain areas of the skin, the vagina, groin, and feet.

Resources

The following organizations and websites provide additional information on boosting your immunity and improving your overall health. Some websites offer nutrition and exercise information, while others provide resources for people who struggle with various immune-related health conditions.

Immune Deficiency

AIDS.gov
aids.gov

AIDS.gov is the U.S. government's official website that communicates about initiatives to combat AIDS and support those who suffer from the illness.

AIDS.org
aids.org

AIDS.org provides education and facilitates an exchange of knowledge as part of its ongoing effort to prevent the spread of HIV and support those who have contracted the virus or AIDS.

Centers for Disease Control and Prevention: HIV/AIDS
cdc.gov/hiv

The HIV/AIDS webpage on the Centers for Disease Control and Prevention (CDC) website is an informative resource for HIV and AIDS patients and medical professionals. Its mission is to provide leadership in helping control the HIV/AIDS epidemic by working with community, state, national, and international partners in surveillance, research, and prevention and evaluation activities.

Immune Deficiency Foundation
primaryimmune.org

The Immune Deficiency Foundation (IDF) provides accurate and timely information for people who have been diagnosed with a primary immunodeficiency disease. The organization helps patients and the medical community through education, outreach, and advocacy programs. It also promotes and funds research to improve treatment options for people suffering from immune deficiency.

INFO4PI.ORG
info4pi.org/aboutPI/index.cfm?section=aboutPI

Primary immunodeficiency affects as many as 1 million Americans and 10 million people worldwide. INFO4PI.ORG helps people with PI and their families learn about the disease and locate medical experts who can help. INFO4PI.ORG also provides resources for medical professionals.

Probiotics and Other Supplements

Medline Plus
nlm.nih.gov/medlineplus/druginformation.html

Medline Plus is a website that helps patients learn more about prescription and over-the-counter drugs, supplements, and herbal remedies.

National Center for Complementary and Alternative Medicine: Oral Probiotics
nccam.nih.gov/health/probiotics/introduction.htm

The Oral Probiotics webpage on the National Center for Complementary and Alternative Medicine (NCCAM) website gives a comprehensive overview of how probiotics can be safely used to improve your health.

National Institutes of Health: Office of Dietary Supplements
ods.od.nih.gov

The Office of Dietary Supplements (ODS) website provides an overview of the vitamins, minerals, and other supplements that support a healthy lifestyle.

Diet

Harvard School of Public Health: Nutrition Source
hsph.harvard.edu/nutritionsource

The Nutrition Source webpage on The Harvard School of Public Health website gives tips for eating right, recommendations on the quantity of different food types and substances that should comprise your diet, and much more.

Nutrition.gov
nutrition.gov

Nutrition.gov is the central hub for information on nutritional guidance and recommendations in the United States. Links are provided to nutrition sites such as choosemyplate.gov, a new government initiative to help educate the public on what type of food is healthy and how much of it to eat.

***SELF*NutritionData**
nutritiondata.self.com

This is a website about nutrition created by *SELF* magazine that offers tools to help you calculate your BMI (body mass index), track your progress, analyze recipes, and find foods by nutrient.

WebMD: Weight Loss & Diet Plans
webmd.com/diet

The Weight Loss & Diet Plans webpage on WebMD offers a useful resource for people who need help losing weight and creating a healthy diet.

Exercise

American Heart Association
heart.org

The American Heart Association's website provides information about getting your heart healthy. It covers topics such as nutrition, fats and oils, fitness, weight management, stress management, smoking cessation, and keeping your kids healthy. Click "Getting Healthy" and explore!

BodyBuilding.com: Exercise Guides
bodybuilding.com/exercises

BodyBuilding.com offers detailed instructions on how to do just about every exercise you can. The site is an invaluable resource whether you're a beginner or someone looking for an encyclopedia on ways to build on the base you already have.

Mayo Clinic: Exercise: 7 Benefits of Regular Physical Activity
mayoclinic.com/health/exercise/HQ01676

The Exercise: 7 Benefits of Regular Physical Activity webpage on the Mayo Clinic's website discusses the seven benefits of regular physical activity, which we discussed in depth in Chapter 7.

WebMD: Fitness & Exercise
webmd.com/fitness-exercise

The Fitness & Exercise webpage on WebMD provides a helpful resource for creating an exercise plan that works for you, as well as a place to get help from the experts.

Stress Management

The American Institute of Stress
stress.org

The American Institute of Stress (AIS) is a comprehensive resource for the latest information related to stress and stress management. AIS can offer referrals and consultations on many stress-related conditions, including posttraumatic stress disorder (PTSD), job-related stress, stress assessment and measurement techniques, and much more.

National Center for Complementary and Alternative Medicine: Meditation
nccam.nih.gov/health/meditation/overview.htm

The Meditation webpage on the National Center for Complementary and Alternative Medicine (NCCAM) website is a solid resource for learning how meditation works, the health benefits of meditation, and how to incorporate meditation into your life.

Psychology Today: **Stress**
psychologytoday.com/basics/stress

The Stress webpage on *Psychology Today* gives information about stress and stress disorders and offers some tools for measuring your own level of stress.

The Transcendental Meditation Program
tm.org

The Transcendental Meditation Program teaches you how to participate in transcendental meditation, one of the simplest and most beneficial forms of the meditation practice. The resources on the site point you in the right direction to get started with your practice.

WebMD: Stress Management Health Center
webmd.com/balance/stress-management

The Stress Management Health Center webpage on WebMD gives you the tools you need to better manage stress, including how to measure, relieve, and avoid it. The site is always being updated with the latest news about stress and your health.

Vaccinations and Hygiene

Centers for Disease Control and Prevention: Vaccines & Immunizations
cdc.gov/vaccines

The Vaccines & Immunizations webpage on the Centers for Disease Control and Prevention (CDC) website provides vaccine schedules for infants, children, and adults, along with descriptions of the diseases that each vaccine immunizes against. The CDC also includes general information about the importance of vaccines and immunizations.

FLU.gov: Vaccinations & Vaccine Safety

flu.gov/prevention-vaccination/vaccination/index.html

The Vaccinations & Vaccine Safety webpage on FLU.gov shows you what you can do about the flu, including what each year's vaccine protects against, how effective the vaccine is that year, and more. FLU.gov also offers a service to locate by ZIP code the flu vaccination clinic nearest to you.

Mayo Clinic: Hand Washing: Do's and Don'ts

mayoclinic.com/health/hand-washing/HQ00407

The Hand Washing: Do's and Don'ts webpage on the Mayo Clinic's website outlines basic protocols for keeping your hands clean and preventing the spread of illness.

Vaccinate Your Baby

vaccinateyourbaby.org

Vaccinate Your Baby separates the myths from the facts about vaccinating babies as proven by research and science. The site provides general information about vaccines and some specifics about vaccine safety.

WellnessFX

wellnessfx.com

WellnessFX is a web-based service that provides access to blood tests, phone consultations to health practitioners, and online data tracking so people can identify and reverse their potential health risks.

Index

A

acai berry, 184-185
acetaminophen, 63
acquired immunodeficiency syndrome (AIDS), 35
active immune memory, 11
adaptive immune system, 4, 9
    cell-mediated immunity, 10
    humoral immunity, 10
    immune memory, 10-11
Addison's disease, 42
adult vaccination boosters, 76
aerobic exercises, 105
age, immunity, 80
AIDS (acquired immunodeficiency syndrome), 35
Airborne, 190-191
airborne illnesses, preventing, 97-98
alcohol, 82
    effects, 84-85
    inflammation, 51
allergens, 38
allergies, 38-39
    food, 43
Almond Butter and Cherry Sandwich, 219

almonds, 174-175
    Almond Butter and Cherry Sandwich, 219
    Chocolate Almond Coconut Balls, 227
ammonia, 95
anaphylaxis, 38-39
antibiotics, 7, 65
    children, 79-80
    detrimental effects, 18
    gastrointestinal infections, 19
    MRSA (Methicillin-resistant Staphylococcus aureus), 23
    natural flora, 180
    strep infections, 28
antibodies, 8-9
antigens, 3-4
antioxidants, 149-150
    sources, 150-151
arsenic, cigarettes, 83
artificial sweeteners, 140-142
aspartame, 141
asthma, 38-40
atherosclerosis, 54, 59-60
attenuated vaccines, 70
autoimmune disease, 41-43
avian flu, 22
azole, 30

E

ear infections, 29-30
echinacea, 186-187
E. coli, 23
eczema, 38-40
elderberry, 185-186
Emergen-C, 191-193
endorphins, 103
energy drinks, 142
Enterococcus faecium, 182
erythrocyte sedimentation rate (ESR), 52
Escherichia coli, 23
ESR (erythrocyte sedimentation rate), 52
estimating caloric needs, 131-132
excessive exercise, 53
exercise, 103
    benefits, 99-103
    creating fitness plans, 103-104
    direct immune response, 101
    excessive, 53
    immune-boosting, 99
    locations, 107-108
    office, 108-109
    overtraining, 109-112
    types, 105-107
expression, genes, 81-82

F

fats, 129, 138-139
    omega-3 fatty acids, 173-174
fiber, beta-glucan, 170
financial stress, 115
fish
    salmon, 173-174
    Seafood Stew, 217

fitness plans, creating, 103-104
flexibility training, 106
flora, 6-7
flu shots, 11
flu vaccines, 72
folic acid, 163
food intolerances, 43
Four-Bean Chili, 215-216
free radicals, 83
Fruit-and-Yogurt Smoothie, 202
Fruit Parfait, 229
fruits, 165
    blueberries, 167
    goji berries, 225
    phytochemicals, 166
    pomegranates, 168-169
fungal infections, 26

G

garlic, 176-177
gastrointestinal (GI) infections, 31
gastrointestinal infections, viral, 19-20
genetic predisposition to hypersensitivities, 40
genetics
    expression, 81-82
    immunity, age, 80
German measles vaccine, 72
ghee, 199
GI (gastrointestinal) infections, 31
GI (glycemic index) score, 135-136
ginseng, 188
globulins, testing, 239
Gluten-Free Walnut-Flax Banana Muffins, 203-204

Chocolate Almond Coconut
Balls, 227
Four-Bean Chili, 215-216
Fruit-and-Yogurt Smoothie,
202
Fruit Parfait, 229
Gluten-Free Walnut-Flax
Banana Muffins, 203-204
Guacamole, 223
Hearty Kale-Sardine Salad,
218
Kim's Chicken Soup, 205-206
Kim's Trail Mix, 225
Lamb Chops and Ratatouille,
211-212
Lentil Soup, 207
Mint-Chocolate Pudding,
230-231
Mixed Berry Crumble, 228
Salmon and Cucumber
Sandwich, 201
Seafood Stew, 217
Steel-Cut Oatmeal with Kiwi,
Banana, and Blueberries, 200
Tangy Skirt Steak and
Tomato-Spinach Salad,
208-209
Tofu Stir-Fry with Wild Rice,
213-214
Vanilla Ice Cream with
Cherries and Pomegranates,
226
Veggie Egg Scramble, 199
Veggie-Filled Acorn Squash,
220
Wasabi Salmon with Sweet
Potato and Brussels Sprouts,
210
White Bean Dip and Carrots,
222

reducing inflammation, 53
reflective meditation, 124
reiki, 37
relaxation
achieving, 119
benefits, 117-118
reproductive tract, 6
respiratory infections, 27-28
respiratory system, 64
respiratory tract, 6
lining, 5
rheumatoid arthritis (RA), 42
riboflavin, 162
risks
heart disease, 55-58
inflammation, 51-52
overtraining, 112
vaccinations, 73-74
weakened immunity, 35-37
rubella vaccine, 72

S

saccharin, 141
Saccharomyces boulardii, 182
salads
Beet, Watermelon, and
Spinach Salad, 224
Hearty Kale-Sardine Salad,
218
Tangy Skirt Steak and
Tomato-Spinach Salad,
208-209
salmon, 173-174
Salmon and Cucumber
Sandwich, 201
Wasabi Salmon with Sweet
Potato and Brussels Sprouts,
210

W-X